P9-DNA-246

The Home Team

The Home Team

Of Mothers, Daughters, and American Champions

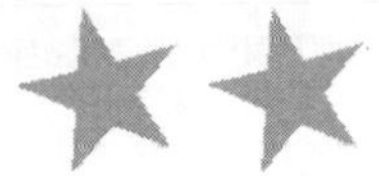

RuthAnn *and* Rebecca Lobo

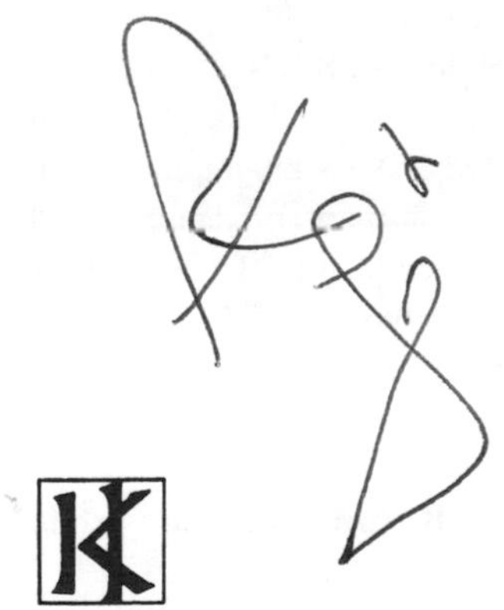

KODANSHA INTERNATIONAL
New York • Tokyo • London

Kodansha America, Inc.
114 Fifth Avenue, New York, New York 10011, U.S.A.

Kodansha International Ltd.
17-14 Otowa 1-chome, Bunkyo-ku, Tokyo 112, Japan

Published in 1996 by Kodansha America, Inc.

Library of Congress Cataloging-in-Publication Data

Lobo, RuthAnn.
The home team : of mothers, daughters, and American champions / RuthAnn and Rebecca Lobo.
p. cm.
ISBN 1-56836-140-8 (HC)
1. Lobo, Rebecca. 2. Lobo, RuthAnn. 3. Women basketball players—United States—Biography. 4. Educators—United States—Biography. 5. Mothers and daughters—United States—Biography. 6. Family—United States. I. Lobo, Rebecca. II. Title.
GV884.L6L63 1996
796.323'092—dc20
[B] 96-6857

Book design by Beehive Production Services

Printed in the United States of America

96 97 98 99 00 BER/B 10 9 8 7 6 5 4 3 2

To Dennis (Dad) whose love allows us to test our wings
To Jason whose gentleness quiets us
To Rachel whose passion ignites us
To God for the gift of each other

Contents

Foreword

I have been asked to pen a few words about "The Great Book" that Rebecca and RuthAnn are writing. (I call it this because when I log onto our PC, this is the title that gains us entry.) RuthAnnie and Becca are just two of the cherished ones of my family life. One, my soulmate, the other my "little-big kid," a term, by the way, that Rebecca detests! To pen lines to be placed in their book is somewhat awkward, like being asked to reminisce at a colleague's testimonial dinner.

I have taken a detached and somewhat dispassionate involvement in the book because this is their undertaking—a written dialogue between mother and daughter. Early on in the proceedings, however, I was asked to proofread a chapter which, as a good husband I did, and I gave my best teacher-hubby opinion. I was met by a somewhat stony stare and a comment, "Well, that's not quite what I had in mind." I have learned in our relationship that some things are better left unsaid and some situations better left untouched. This book was one of them.

I will assume the readers will develop a mind-picture of the rest of the Lobo family from whatever RuthAnn and Rebecca have written and, coupled with whatever unflattering photos make it into the book, will draw their own conclusions.

Suffice it to say that I am immensely proud of all my near and extended family. I feel triply blessed with great parents, a loving wife, and three terrific children. Sit back and enjoy the book. Chuckle, smile, shed some tears, or nod your head in agreement.

Welcome to Lobo-land and God bless!

Den Lobo
December 1995

Acknowledgments

We would like to express our sincere gratitude for the support and encouragement of friends and colleagues throughout the writing of this book. We thank our agent and friend, Kenton Edelin, for his many hours of work on our behalf. We also would like to express our appreciation to the staff at Kodansha America for their painstaking work in bringing this book to completion. We are especially grateful to our editor, Deborah Baker, whose patience, guidance, humor, and personal commitment turned a dream into a reality. Finally, we would like to thank our extended family whose unconditional love nurtures, comforts, and strengthens us in all our endeavors.

★ 1 ★

A Girl and a Ball

★ REBECCA

I've taken this drive a million times. It's early summer and I'm heading home from my new apartment near the University of Connecticut campus in Storrs. Finals ended about three weeks ago, but it seems longer than that. The day after my last exam, I flew to Colorado to try out for the USA National Team, the core of the women's basketball team that will compete in the Atlanta Olympics a little over a year from now. I didn't even have time to pack up my dorm room before leaving. My mom came down and cleared out everything that was there. After surviving the cut, I had twenty-four hours at home, time only to do laundry and sleep before leaving for a European tour. After two weeks overseas I came back for one night to pack my things again and move into my apartment at school. This road is like an old friend.

Most people move away from home for the first time when they go off to college. They have to deal with saying good-bye to their parents, high school sweetheart, and best friends. Since UConn was only an hour from my house and I didn't have a boyfriend in high school, I didn't have to deal with all the emotion that comes with leaving home for the first time. I knew people at school, I knew the area, and I knew my family was only an hour away. Although I never went home on the weekends, I could have. If I had a problem, I knew my mom would take a quick spin up to school and take me out to dinner (she did this more than once). My security blanket stretched easily from Southwick to Storrs.

That was not the only reason I chose to go to UConn, though I'm sure it entered into my decision. Similarly, when it came time to graduate, there were a number of reasons behind my decision to stay on in Storrs, if only for one last summer. I had a bunch of appearances to make in Connecticut, plus I needed to use UConn's rehab facilities after undergoing arthroscopic surgery on my knee. The fact that my boyfriend was going to be in Storrs was no small consideration either. So there was really never any question where I would spend the summer.

This visit home is nothing special—an appointment with the dentist, grab a few things from my room. The drive has become so routine that I can almost do it with my eyes closed. The only thing that makes this trip a little more special is that I'm in my new car. It's the first automobile I have ever owned. In high school and college I had bugged my parents for a car constantly. My brother and sister had use of a family car, but by the time I was old enough to drive I had to make do with rides to school from friends (thanks Nathan!) since my brother needed the extra car at law school. A few times I even tried to tell my parents that I *deserved* one because I had gotten a college scholarship. No reply.

I went through different phases. At one point I was in love with the Mazda Miata (though I never would have fit!), then I wanted a Jeep Wrangler. For the most part, however, I didn't care. I dropped hints all the time until my mom finally said, "We would get you a car in a second if we could afford to." Then I thought about my parents' expenses, which included my brother's Dartmouth education and my sister's school loans—not to mention the fact that my parents' credit card bills are always sky high because my sister and I love to be taken clothes shopping. So I waited until I graduated from college. In exchange for doing a car commercial for the Connecticut

Chevy dealerships, I got a great deal on a 1995 Blazer that I love (shameless plug).

On this trip home, I take the same roads as always. Route 195, then I-84 to 91. Just across the Connecticut border is Southwick, Massachusetts, the small town where I've lived almost all my life. Finally, I turn onto my street and drive two miles down a road lined with trees until I reach the family driveway.

A driveway that seems to shrink with each year that passes.

A driveway that started as pebbles and is now asphalt.

A driveway that has had more basketballs bounced on its surface, bikes skidded over it, and skateboards ridden over its bumps than any one person can imagine.

A driveway that was my whole world while I was growing up. I am home.

* * * *

People ask me how I started playing basketball. It's not a fairy tale. It's simply the story of a young girl who loved to stand in her driveway and shoot a rubber ball through a basketball hoop. I don't remember how old I was when the hoop was put up. I don't remember if I fell in love with the game right away. I simply remember standing in the driveway and shooting for hours at a time. I remember playing alone, playing with my brother and sister, playing with my parents. It was more than a game to me. It was a chance to escape and to dream.

Sometimes I played because I wanted to get out of a bad mood, sometimes because I was worried about an upcoming test. Sometimes playing basketball was just a great way to forget myself. When I stepped out into the driveway, I was no longer Rebecca Lobo. I was Larry Bird or I was Dr. J. But often I was no one and would just let my thoughts take me where they wanted to go. I would shoot the ball toward the hoop unconsciously, as if I were in a trance. I didn't have any parents coaching me or pressuring me to practice shooting or dribbling; I could do what I wanted out there. Maybe that's why I loved it so much. It was the one place I could go as a kid and do whatever I pleased. It was a way of being alone but better than just idly sitting around, which I hated.

During my four years at UConn I left my family driveway behind for Gampel Pavilion. Gampel is UConn's basketball arena—it's a big dome with doors all around and whether you enter or just look in from the outside, all you can see is the scoreboard and the bleachers. Because I know the place inside and out, it's more like a house than a sports arena to me (a very big, rent-free house). After my freshman year, I knew where everything was and I felt as comfortable hanging out on the couches in the team's lounge watching TV as I did in my living room back home. I couldn't possibly count the number of hours I spent shooting baskets there. I spent way more time there than in my dorm room.

During the summers I usually took classes and lived at school so I could get ahead in my courses and take fewer credit hours during the basketball season. Since there were not many people on campus then, I headed over to Gampel in the morning to shoot hoops. And just like that driveway at home, there I discovered a world all my own. As the sun came up, the light coming through the doors grew in intensity until the whole space was flooded with brightness. It was air conditioned to just the right degree. The emptiness of the court on these mornings provided me with a comfort zone I have not been able to find anywhere else in my life. The men's team took the court in the afternoon, but I had it all to myself every morning. When you're by yourself dribbling the ball, all you hear is the rhythm of the ball hitting the wooden floor. When a shot hits the rim hard, the sound is loud and shocking. In order to maintain a sense of peace you try hard to swish every shot.

Gampel couldn't be more different during games. You hear the fans, your coach on the sidelines, your teammates, the ball, the sneakers squeaking on the floor. You smell popcorn, nachos, pizza, and other "healthy" foods. The place comes alive. When you're there alone, you're no longer on stage. With the bleachers pushed back, you're in the middle of a huge empty space.

Just as my shots traveled toward the basket, my mind traveled to many different places, imagining many different possibilities. Problems and worries disappeared. If I was excited about something, I became calm. If I was moody, I might begin to feel sad. This wasn't a sadness I was trying to escape from, but an emotion I could work through. I let my mind wander, exploring my highest hopes, my secret dreams. Sometimes I fantasized about winning the national championship or bending down to have an Olympic gold medal placed around my neck.

More often than not, however, I thought about things completely unrelated to basketball. I thought of ways to resolve small conflicts. If my parents were coming up for a game and wanted to take me out to dinner, but I wanted to join my friends and teammates for dinner instead, I had to figure out how to tell my parents in a way that wouldn't hurt their feelings. I played out the possible conversations in my head. Other times I just daydreamed about lying on the beach or hanging out with my friends. By the time my thoughts returned to Gampel, usually an hour or more had passed.

Sometimes people came onto the court to talk to me. Football players often stopped by after working out in the weight room and, seeing me through the glass windows in the gym, would come in and say, "Let's play one on one," or "Let's play horse." I wanted to say, "No, leave me alone," but I never did. I didn't want to be rude and knew they just wanted to have fun; people who don't play basketball just love to shoot around. So they would shoot and I would rebound for them and we would talk. Eventually they would leave and I'd get back to my own thing. Usually I didn't mind, but sometimes it drove me crazy; I don't think they ever realized that they were pulling me back from another world. They never imagined what was going through my head or what was filling my heart. But I could never bring myself to say, "Leave me alone, I'm daydreaming."

Once classes resumed in the fall and students and fellow teammates returned to campus, it was much more difficult to find time alone on the court. No one understood why I enjoyed this time alone so much and I never tried to explain. For the most part, I kept my thoughts to myself. That quiet time alone on the court kept me sane during some of the crazier times of my career.

I imagine enjoying the court alone started when I was younger. I often misplaced my house key and had to wait for my mother to get home. The time flew by if I shot hoops in the driveway, like the day in fifth grade when I got into trouble at school for sending a note around the room about the substitute teacher. The note said, "Mrs. M. has a mustache." I had never done anything like that before. I might have said something under my breath, but I had never before passed a note around (I was a little smartass, but I don't think I was cruel). Unfortunately, the teacher found the note and recognized my handwriting. She sent me to the principal's office. I didn't feel too bad about that—I felt bad because of the look on the teacher's face when she confronted me with the little slip of paper. I could tell I had hurt her feelings, and I felt terrible. I left school with a note from the principal explaining what I had done—a note that needed to be signed by my "legal guardian" and returned the next day.

I knew that I was going to get into trouble and thoughts of various punishments floated around in my head on the way home from school. I wished that I was good at forging my father's name like my sister Rachel was. She had perfected it. (Then again, she needed to. She got into a lot more trouble than I did.) Even if I could have, I'm sure I would have been too afraid of getting caught to try it. As I waited for my mom to get home, I shot baskets. I must have been shooting around for an hour or so before she pulled up, went into the house, and unloaded the groceries. I followed her in with the note. I remember standing in the kitchen watching her read it. My punishment never came. Instead, my mom just looked at me and told me that what I had written was very cruel. She signed the letter and gave it back to me. Perhaps that incident is still so vivid because I learned that day that sometimes you can learn a lesson better when you are not punished than when you are.

It was also the first time I remember using basketball as a way of coping. While I was shooting in my driveway that afternoon, I managed to forget about what I had done and that I would be punished. I forgot about the look on the substitute teacher's face. I forgot about the principal's office and about the note that needed to be signed. Looking back, the note was not that big a deal; the ability to work through difficulties was. Many people, particularly young kids, need some way to handle the pain or anxiety, however small or profound, in their lives. Basketball became my way.

Later, when I was a junior in college, some reporter wrote about how I had considered quitting basketball when my mother told me about her breast cancer. The thought had never even crossed my mind! I almost laughed when I read that in her article. I wonder if the reporter would understand if I told her that basketball was what had saved me during that time. I wonder if she could comprehend the fact that practicing or playing was the only time I could completely free my mind of everything that was going on; that my mom's illness would not enter my mind at all as long as I was on the court playing this simple game.

I doubt the reporter, or anyone else for that matter, could ever know what basketball meant to me my junior year. It relieved me of my worries except those that arose on the court. I prayed for my mom, I cared for my mom, but I didn't focus on what she must have been feeling. I didn't want to add to her worries. Instead, I concentrated on the next game or the next practice and not on how she would feel after the next chemotherapy treatment. I made my biggest problem or concern our last loss or our next victory.

Later, when I was a senior, I felt guilty. I told myself that I hadn't thought about what she was going through as much as I should have. I had let myself get wrapped up in my own world of basketball. But basketball, unlike real life, allowed me to have problems and goals I had control over. Nothing that I did back then, short of praying, could affect my mother's battle with her cancer. I couldn't make the disease win or lose. I couldn't make her blood cells do this or do that. But I could make the ball go into the basket. I could have an effect on our team's efforts to win and not lose. I could do *something*. As a result, I put most of my energy into an arena where I could make a difference.

And, for however brief a time, my mother also left her worries at the gate when she watched us play that spring. When I was out there on the court with my mom in the stands, we both thought about nothing but the game. Just like those precious summer days when I was all alone on the court at Gampel Pavilion, I let my mind go free. Free of the problems I had. Free of the problems my mom had. Free of everything that was out of my control. I felt like a kid again.

A kid in her driveway shooting baskets without a care in the world.

A kid whose biggest problem was giving her mom a note from the principal.

A kid whose dream was to grow up and play ball with the Boston Celtics.

Sometimes I wish I was back in that driveway, just a girl with a ball and a dream. Sometimes, when I pick up a ball, that wish comes true.

★ 2 ★

Laughing Until We Cry

★ RUTHANN

My husband Dennis grew up in the industrial city of New Britain, Connecticut, amid smokestacks and the sounds of city life. Not long after we moved to Southwick, Massachusetts, he looked at me and remarked, "It's really dark outside." I thought this a most peculiar statement. "Of course it's dark outside," I said, looking at him oddly. "It's nighttime!" "But," he said, "it's *really* dark." It wasn't until this conversation had been repeated several times that I realized he had grown up under the glare of street lights and for him, it really was *really* dark outside. In Medfield, Massachusetts, when I grew up, dark at night was normal.

Southwick is a small town. Twenty years ago, when we first moved here, the population was under ten thousand, the school system was excellent, and town meetings afforded the citizenry their say in everything from a new school roof to roadside stands. The road to our house had been paved only within the past ten years or so, and it meandered between densely wooded areas, open meadows, and fields. The houses were few and not one was within earshot of another.

Wrapped in the solitude of our new surroundings, my husband and children—Jason (age 8), Rachel (age 4), and Rebecca (age 2)—quickly grew accustomed to the sights and sounds of the country living I had known as a child: the chatter of the tree toads marking the arrival of spring, the throaty croak of bullfrogs in summer, the flicker of evening fireflies in the backyard. Our family car often stopped for those hapless box turtles found trudging from one side of the road to the other, with one or the other of us jumping out to help it across. To "see if the deer kids are out," Dennis slowed down in front of the pasture down the road, with an eye out for the family of deer that grazed there. Not too far from the house was a tiny pond whose lively ecosystem can, in part, be credited to our family. From a nearby fishing hole, Den and the children caught, by hook or bucket, catfish and shiners, pollywogs and frogs, to deposit there. Armed with handfuls of bread, our kids cultivated the life in that pond for years.

There is something to be said about living in an area where nothing is within walking distance. Our family grew up relying on each other for company. Lacking any landscaping sense, we transformed our yard into a playing field. After dinner Wiffle ball and basketball games were endless. Mastering the art of bike riding did not take much time for our children, and it was not long before there were bike paths throughout our yard. After graduating from Big Wheels, the kids took up sporty little numbers with banana seats. For years the kids zipped among the trees and over the bumps they had so arduously created.

Long before the inside of our home was finished, our backyard featured an above-ground swimming pool. Relatives thought that our priorities were out of whack; after all, we only had rough flooring in the master bedroom. That pool, however, brought the family more pleasure than any wall-to-wall carpeting could have. It saw hours of use each day of the summer. The kids jumped, splashed, and created a number of competitive events among themselves. The screen door creaked open with regularity as little wet feet dripped back and forth across the kitchen to the bathroom. Three pairs of blue lips shuddered above worn out towels. Den and I were called on to watch new dives, judge underwater races, and give piggyback rides in the water. Blessed were the few moments when I had the pool to myself and could float about without being pounced on.

Sadly, few children today grow up in the safety and wonder of the country. Hours once spent roaming through fields or fishing have been replaced by the electronic beeps and gurgles of video and computer games. Two or three mile walks to a friend's house are fraught by the increasing danger that pervades even the most stable of communities. The freedom once enjoyed by our children is gone; they have become ensnared in a web of commercial exploitation and the fear of strangers.

Despite the rustic setting, however, we were not the Waltons. I learned early in my marriage, and was reminded every fall with the opening of the football season, that the New York Giants took precedence over just about everything, including dinner. I should have taken a cue from my mother-in-law, who always served dinner before the onset of the game. My loyalty to the New England Patriots notwithstanding, I found myself engaged in a private war of sabotage as I refused to plan my life around football. My dinners were frequently ready at the same time the games started. I refused to fuss with meals unless full attention was given to enjoying them. I cheered for the Washington Redskins. "I didn't know you were a Redskins' fan," Dennis once observed. "I'm not," I replied, "I'm just cheering for any team who is competing against the New York Giants!"

Unlike football, I suppose, marriage is not about making or keeping score. I learned not only to enjoy football more but to include important games in our weekend schedule. Den in return became less frenetic about seeing every minute of every game. His love of the sport rubbed off on our children, and I still marvel at their early understanding of the game and knowledge of the players. Long before Rebecca could read, she could rattle off the names of the players on both the Giants and Patriots teams, and she understood the plays as they happened. Spontaneous football games after dinner on the front lawn were the order of the day.

Other games kept us busy too. We played Hide and Seek and London Bridge. Rachel was desperate to be the cheese when we played The Farmer in the Dell. There she would be, ecstatic in the middle of our tiny circle, as the rest of us sang aloud, "And the cheese stands alone." Board games filled cold winter evenings as we slowly graduated from Candyland and Trouble to Boggle, Scrabble, and Trivial Pursuit. The word games were always my favorite, whereas Dennis was the master at Trivial Pursuit. My husband, the history teacher, has an incredible knack for storing and retrieving information in his head. Competitive from the start, the kids picked their teams accordingly; Mom for vocabulary and Dad for the details. For those more contemplative and quiet evenings, there was The Sock Game. We gathered in the living room wearing socks but no shoes, and the object was to remove the socks of anybody and everybody else without losing our own. I'm not sure we ever had a winner. I do remember five people getting silly, shrieking hysterically, and rolling about on the living room floor.

Bedtime was story time in our house, which meant cuddling around the fire with pajama-clad kids sprawled on our laps, or piled together on the family recliner. Den or I read books from our childhood, as well as Dr. Seuss and the Berenstain Bears. Den resurrected his tattered and worn copy of *Uncle Wiggley's Adventures*, complete with his childhood scribbles. To this day when we are about to embark on something new, Den will say, "Well, we're about to have an Uncle

Wiggley adventure." My favorites were Mother Goose rhymes. I always found time to read or recite nursery rhymes. Winnie the Pooh was another family member. With children clinging to the sides of the recliner, we would giggle over Eeyore's missing tail and Pooh's insatiable appetite for honey.

* * * *

Although we have lived in Southwick, Massachusetts, for twenty years, Rebecca was born in Connecticut and lived the first two years of her life in the Nutmeg State. My husband and I have worked in Granby, Connecticut, forever, and all three of our children attended Valley Preschool there. To complicate matters of where our loyalty lies, a good portion of Southwick juts into Connecticut and there is much conjecture as to how this bit of Massachusetts property invaded the border of its neighbor to the south.

This geographical oddity would probably have remained a bit of trivia over wine and cheese had it not been for the success of the UConn women in the spring of 1995. As Rebecca and her team advanced from victory to victory, the locals from both states, but the border towns in particular, suddenly began to argue over who had the right to claim Rebecca as their own. One editorial in the *Hartford Courant* suggested a militant uprising to confiscate and reclaim Southwick as part of Connecticut. At the very least, the editors insisted, a reconfiguration of the border was needed in order to change our address from one state to the other.

Driving home from work one afternoon, I chuckled as I listened to a Hartford radio station solicit opinions from listeners about annexing Southwick for the state of Connecticut. Referring to the *Courant* editorial, the talk show host queried, "Her heart is in Connecticut. Shouldn't her abode be there too?" I laughed out loud as he randomly called Chuck's Steak House in Southwick to raise the question, "What would it take to make Southwick a part of Connecticut?"

The debate continued in a local store in Southwick where I stopped to get a newspaper. One customer told me how excited everyone at his place of work in Granby was because "*both* Mr. and Mrs. Lobo worked in Granby public schools." With a proprietarial air, he recounted how he had reminded his coworkers that Rebecca's roots and her address were in Southwick. He was indignant that anyone would even consider Rebecca anything but a Southwick hero. I acknowledged his sentiments with a smile and caught myself chuckling again as I made my way home.

Some time after the University of Connecticut women's basketball team had won the NCAA National Championship in Minneapolis, Minnesota, I rode with my husband to the local recycling station to dispose of the week's bottles, cans, and paper. Displayed outside a small brick commercial building that we passed was a large sign announcing, "Congratulations Rebecca Lobo! 1995 National Player of the Year!" I had driven by that and countless similar signs around Southwick. Somehow, however, for the first time since the final buzzer sounded at the Final Four announcing that indeed the UConn Huskies were the national champions, the full impact of my daughter's accomplishments truly hit me.

I suddenly felt an overwhelming sense of pride and emotion quite beyond anything I had ever felt before. My eyes filled with tears and my throat tightened as I looked at my husband. "Reading that sign," I whispered hoarsely, "has brought home to me the reality of what Rebecca has accomplished. I've told reporters hundreds of times how wonderful it all is, but this is the first time it has actually struck me. And the people in our hometown feel that pride as well." Suddenly, I began to make some sense of the fuss and the clamor that surrounded us in the aftermath of victory.

By her senior year, there were few places Rebecca could travel unnoticed. By the Final Four there were few places my husband and I could travel unnoticed. I watched in wonder as people from young children to senior citizens waited patiently in line for hours to touch this child of mine, to exchange stories, to offer a small gift or secure an autograph. Her father and I returned home from each visit with arms full of the photographs, drawings, stuffed animals, flowers, and handmade crafts people so generously showered on our daughter. I am still in awe of the love affair that blossomed between the public and Rebecca. People lingered after games in hope of catching her attention for a moment. We heard from many parents how much she inspired their children to work hard both in school and on the basketball court.

"My child is Rebecca's biggest fan," was a frequent comment.

"Photographs of your daughter are all over my child's bedroom wall. What a wonderful role model she is," went another.

"I really don't care if my daughter has a role model or not," one reporter who prides himself on unbiased coverage of sports gruffly confided, "but after sitting and chatting with Rebecca, my daughter has announced that Rebecca is her friend. So I guess if she wants to have Rebecca as her role model, it's okay with me."

We always marveled at those statements because we still remember that little girl whose bedroom overflowed with stuffed animals, notes from friends, and trinkets won at carnivals that she couldn't throw away; that little girl who dallied at bedtime and who balked at taking her cough syrup.

I will always remember the faces of the fans. Wearing everything from hats covered with bone-shaped doggie biscuits to earrings made from tiny basketballs, they gushed enthusiasm and told war stories of icy roads traveled and dinners missed for the sake of UConn women's basketball games. I think I loved best the over-sixty crowd whose ruddy complexions were dead give-aways of impassioned battles with the referees. Eyes sparkling as another victory had been tucked to bed, they clustered on the mezzanine at Gampel, rehashed each play, and delighted in evaluating the officials' performance. Occasionally, on away trips, these very fans would discover themselves in the same hotel as the officials. Returning after the game, weary officials would find themselves explaining the role of the referee and the rules of the game until late into the night.

I remember, too, watching Rebecca learn to handle this adoration. There was a young boy, a street kid from Hartford, brought to a game by his social worker. When I introduced him to Rebecca after the game, he was speechless, paralyzed with awe. "Come over here," she said. Putting her arm around his shoulder, she asked about his interests. When he offered a quiet question, she whispered an answer in his ear. He continued to simply gaze at her. It was obvious he felt like the most important person in Gampel Pavilion. I witnessed this and scenes similar to it repeatedly. To see my daughter, not long out of childhood herself, reach out to a young boy and identify his worth as a human being was a scene I will always keep in my heart.

No one in our family was born into celebrity and the sudden attention focused on Rebecca during her college years was unfamiliar to us. I've always insisted, however, that had my mother, Ruth Caroline Sauer, been born at a different place under other circumstances, she could easily have found her image on the silver screen. Pictures from her late teens and early twenties reveal a sensual beauty reminiscent of the movie stars of the forties. She had dark, flirtatious eyes and wore her brown hair rolled up on the sides in a style typical of the times. Add to her coquettish pose an iron will and a touch of spitfire, and there emerges a young woman who was courted and wooed by many. One young man who sought her heart and hand left in tears when Mom told him she couldn't see him anymore because they were cousins (about twenty times removed). Another suitor bought her a hope chest and filled it with pots and pans. "I hope they all burn if you don't marry me," he uttered, a wish that was later fulfilled when she married someone else. The love of her life, however, was more casual in his pursuit, a clever tactic with a woman who was used to getting her way.

Jimmy McLaughlin was a handsome, strapping 6'5" Irishman with crystal blue eyes and curly blonde hair. He first spotted my mother as she shook carpets from the back porch of her house. He confided to a friend, "That's the woman I'm going to marry." Like his future bride, he too was accustomed to the attention and attraction of the opposite sex. It is not surprising that, after being introduced to her, he not only wanted but expected to be the central figure in her life. On one weekend trip home from the Army Air Corps, he waited until Sunday to contact her. Not to be taken lightly, Mom made sure that another man she was dating was on hand when Jimmy McLaughlin paid a call. "Jimmy," she said, "I'd like you to meet my fiancé." The next time Jimmy came home on leave, he carried with him an engagement ring.

At an age younger than Rebecca is now, my mother became a sweetheart, wife, mother, and widow. She married her good-looking Irishman and, like so many women of the time, kissed him good-bye as he prepared to defend his country. His flight overseas was delayed when engine trouble forced a layover in Maine. My mother joined him for what would be their last time together. That union resulted in my conception, a fact that delighted my father who loved children. Two months later, on June 22, 1943, the plane Jimmy McLaughlin rode as tail gunner was shot down over Huls, Germany. Four of the five crewmen came home at war's end; one did not. My mother received the following letter:

My Darling Wife,

Dearest, this is quite a complicated letter to write, but I'll try to explain to the best of my ability.

This is supposed to be a last word to our loved ones in case we are one of the unfortunate in this horrible war.

Darling, if you should ever get this letter, which I hope you don't, it won't mean that I've actually died unless it's confirmed as such by the government. We may be just held as prisoners—so don't give up hope, my baby snooks.

Darling, tell our baby that his or her daddy regrets not ever seeing him or her. I know it will be the sweetest baby in all the world, because its mother is the sweetest girl in the world.

Darling, I love you more than you could ever know. That's from the bottom of my heart. I loved you since the first day I laid my eyes on you.

Your loving husband,

Jimmy

I'll close hoping you never have the opportunity of opening this letter. All my things will be sent to you. I love you. Be a good girl, baby. Gee I love you too much.

* * * *

Years later, when I first saw my father's letter, I turned it over to find the words "I love you" scrawled repeatedly in my mother's handwriting. I never asked when her words were written, but I suspect it was during her darkest and loneliest despair.

Raising a child single-handed is never easy for anyone and is especially difficult when coupled with grief. Luckily, my mother grew up with nine brothers and one sister. There was little money for luxuries but their home was rich in laughter and love, and home was where she returned after my father's death. For the first year and a half of my life, I was spoiled by a host of aunts and uncles who took me for walks, bought me toys, and played with me endlessly.

At some point, however, my maternal grandmother sent my mother off without me for a few days vacation. While traveling on a trolley in Philadelphia with my Aunt Flossie, my mother found herself engaged in a conversation with a wiry, dark-eyed Merchant Marine with tightly curled hair and a boyish grin. He and his friends accompanied my mom and aunt to the Philadelphia Zoo, and correspondence between my mom and him began. A romance developed via the U.S. mail and it was through letters that Roger Hardy first learned about me. Arriving one day earlier than expected, he found my mother scrubbing floors on her hands and knees and me needing a diaper change. Without flinching, he lovingly swooped me up in his arms and my mom knew that she would give her heart away again.

After my mother's remarriage, we moved to Massachusetts although we still journeyed to Wilkes Barre, Pennsylvania, to visit my mother's family each summer. My grandparents' house sat at the crest of a hill and was separated from neighboring homes by a narrow margin of space. A large porch swept around two sides, and it was always here I first spotted my grandfather, seated with his newspaper, upon our arrival. With his glasses nestled on the tip of his nose, he peered over at me with affection. He took me with him on the trolley, a real treat for a country kid, and together we purchased steamers by the bushel to enjoy for dinner the following evening. He introduced me to liverwurst sausage and Lebanon bologna. He was married to the woman I loved with all my heart.

Like my grandfather, Grandma was of German heritage. She was short and stout, her hair was gray, her eyes a warm brown, and her left cheek bore a rose petal birthmark. Soft and round, her body had borne eleven children and suffered three miscarriages. Grandma was a baker and a seamstress. Though she lived by the rod of a taskmistress, her eyes sometimes betrayed her. "RuthAnn!" she'd yell. "Get up! You're sleeping your life away. Get up you lazy lump!" Rattled to the core, I'd jump out of bed, tumble downstairs, and head for the kitchen. Seeing the wash already on the line and the wringer machine in its place, I'd be certain that breakfast had long since been put away. Chagrined that Grandma considered me a slacker, I'd slump into my chair and look guiltily at the clock—7 A.M.!

Grandma represented strict order: three meals a day at seven, noon, and five. Laundry was done religiously on Monday and ironed on Tuesday. The porch, sidewalk, and kitchen floor were scrubbed every Saturday after the baking was done. On Sunday the air was filled with the aroma of chicken baking in the coal stove.

My tasks, performed with few complaints, included dish washing, table setting, bed making, sweeping, and filling the coal scuttle. Sometimes I was entrusted with the errands to a nearby market. My wages were bountiful: handmade dresses, pretzels from a tin atop the refrigerator, a Creamsicle in early evening, or a trip to the five-and-dime for a three-scoop banana split. On one particularly hot afternoon, Grandma shared a can of beer with me, pouring it in a teacup in case my parents arrived home early. If I prodded her enough, she would recite an off-color playground jingle.

Hallelujah, ride a donkey,
Hallelujah, pull its hair,
Hallelujah, lift its tail up
And see what is there!

She would then clap her hands on her belly and shake with laughter. Wiping the tears from her eyes with her apron, she would shoo me on to other things and her formidable manner would return.

Grandma died during my pregnancy with Rebecca. On my last visit I sat by her side and let her know that another baby was due. She couldn't speak, but the glisten in her eye told me she understood. Rebecca's middle name is Rose after Grandma.

Another legacy, however unlikely, of this stoic grandmother was the strain of pure silliness that runs in my family. One summer, Grandma told my steady boyfriend that just like my Uncle Carl, she enjoyed smoking cigars in private. Sneaking around the side of the house, my father took him to peek in the window. There sat Grandma pretending to smoke a large cigar. Said my boyfriend, "I wouldn't have believed it if I hadn't seen it with my own eyes." My aunts and uncles, now in their seventies, remain inveterate pranksters. Uncle Ralphie, my mother's "baby" brother, has insisted on calling Dennis "Geppetto" ever since Den grew his mustache some twenty-odd years ago. One recent Christmas he sent Den a Pinocchio cup with a tag addressed to "Dad" from "Son." For years the family held reunions in Pennsylvania attended by aunts, uncles, and dozens of cousins with their offspring from as far away as Washington state. While Uncle Harry performed his magic tricks and cousin Jeannette sang her Christian medley, Uncle Ralphie ran about with sparkling space antennae on his head.

My mother is equally excessive. She thought nothing one summer of meeting her brother's boss dressed in brogans, a house dress, and fake eyes plastered next to her nose while her hair covered her real eyes. Upon meeting my husband-to-be for the first time, she sported a blonde wig, black velvet Capri pants with matching top, and introduced herself as my sister. Now in her seventies, she still disguises herself at Halloween and awaits unsuspecting trick-or-treaters. She once dressed up as a troll, using a long coat to hide the fact that she was on bended knees and had my father's shoes sitting in front of her. My brother overheard one departing trick or treater tell another that Mr. Hardy was married to one ugly woman.

Den's wit is entirely unappreciated, met only with groans and rolling eyes. It is he who dubbed the kids with nicknames forever immortalized on lunch bags, in notes, and on tee shirts. Jason, for whatever reason, was called Pear, Piggly Pear, and Piggly. One evening long ago, while the family was watching Jason play baseball at the Southwick Rec Center, a small boy asked three-year-old Rebecca who she was cheering for.

"My brother," she responded.

"What's your brother's name?" queried the boy.

"Jason," she said.

"Jason what?" pursued the young inquisitor.

"Jason Piggly!"

Rachel's nickname was Miss Fish. She not only had a great fondness for fishing, she also transported the greatest amount of bread from my kitchen to feed the fish in the pond. Her sister was lovingly known as the Beccaphant because "Beccaphants never forget." Den would say within her hearing, "Uh oh, Granny Goose is coming. Oops! Don't tell her I said that!" As soon as my mother arrived, Becca would run to the door and soberly proclaim, "Granny, guess what Daddy called you!" It was also unwise to offhandedly promise or suggest anything within Rebecca's earshot because she held you to it. One night she physically transformed herself into the Beccaphant by attaching a long stocking to her nose and swaying it back and forth as she entered the living room. Even I have fallen victim to my husband's penchant for nicknames. As a very little girl, I was known as the Keyhole Peeker for having once been caught peeking in the bathroom keyhole while my Uncle Carl was in there. To Den, however, I will always be known as the Couchopotomus in honor of my fondness for snoozing on the couch.

Horseplay, tickle attacks, and shared copies of Far Side cartoons have kept laughter in the house. Once, in response to my fishing for a compliment on one of my suppers, Den and the kids held their arms out straight, clapped their hands in unison, and made loud barking noises. This became our family's official "Seal of Approval." And then there is the daily race to the mailbox to collect the day's delivery. It sounds absurd, but as soon as we hear the mail carrier, Den and I try to sneak past each other out of the house and dash to the mailbox. I have been known to announce a false phone call in order to get a head start out the door. As we run side by side down the driveway, pulling on each other's shirts to slow the other down, we laugh so hard we can barely stumble forward.

I have noticed, however, that what my children find funny, even hysterical, within the privacy of the family home does not travel well past the mailbox. From my experience as a counselor and a parent, I am keenly aware that once kids reach adolescence, they are convinced that all eyes follow them wherever they go. Their greatest fear is that they will be seen with a hair out of place, an outfit that doesn't match, or an embarrassing parent. A barely discernible blemish becomes a reflecting beacon that flashes the message "Look at me! Look at me!" My general response to all of this is "Nobody is going to notice!"

The kids are quick to remind me that "Nobody is going to notice" is full of exceptions. The fact that members of our family range in height from 5'10" to 6'11" doesn't help us elude interested onlookers. This first became apparent to me when I talked the girls into accompanying me one summer evening to a local stand for ice cream cones. I assured them that no one would see that they were in their pajamas; they could, I said, wait in the car while I bought the ice cream. Unfortunately, our car was rear-ended as I turned into the parking lot of the ice cream stand, and the news of the Lobo family fender bender traveled quickly on private scanners in living rooms all over town. The girls were horrified as the police, ambulance, and interested bystanders rallied around our vehicle in an effort to help as well as satisfy their curiosity about our bedtime wear.

As a parent, however, I have learned to work this anxiety to my advantage. On one Christmas shopping spree with the girls and several of their friends, I grew tired and announced it was time to head for home. To my dismay the girls dilly-dallied and kept weaving their way throughout the stores en route to our exit. In desperation and in keeping with the holiday spirit, I burst into song as I kept pace behind them. Mortified and wanting to escape any further embarrassment, they scurried ahead as I successfully herded them out the door.

Humor and the threat of embarrassment are also neglected, but often effective, disciplinary tools at school as well. I am referring to that sort of embarrassment that occurs when teases and good-natured pranks are done affectionately, even lovingly; I am not referring to the kind of humiliation that destroys a child's self-image and crushes the soul. I had a young chatterbox in one of my classes who found himself in detention with me one afternoon. For thirty minutes I serenaded him with improvised lyrics sung to the tune of a renowned American musical.

Hel-lo Russell, well hel-lo Russell, it's so nice to have you after school with me. . . .

When the detention period had elapsed, my pet made a hasty retreat and future disciplinary actions were forestalled by the mere humming of the tune. He always responded in open-eyed horror and swiftly buttoned lips.

I learned a lot from my family.

★ 3 ★

Tomboy

★ *REBECCA*

I remember the first and only time I wrote to the president of the United States. I was in the fifth grade at the time and I sent a letter to Ronald Reagan. I have no idea what I said to him (he probably didn't either); it was just one of those assignments popular with fifth grade teachers. I didn't even know what a political party was or what the parties stood for (I now wonder if the politicians know). I was not one of those kids who stood up and said that someday I was going to be the president of the United States. Nevertheless, even at that age, I believed I could become whatever I wanted to become.

I had, what seemed to me, good reason to believe this. One Christmas when I was little I asked for a tool belt. I don't know what my fascination was with being a carpenter, but I was obsessed with that one gift. I got it. My parents didn't seem to have an opinion about what toys were or were not appropriate. My sister Rachel and I even received football uniforms for Christmas one year, because I was convinced that one day I would be good enough to play for the New England Patriots or the New York Giants. Santa obviously supported the idea.

Or, I wanted to play basketball for the Boston Celtics. When I was in the third grade, I wrote the following letter to their general manager:

Dear Mr. Auerbach,

I really like watching the Celtics play. You do a really good job. I want you to know that I am going to be the first girl to play for the Boston Celtics.

Rebecca Lobo

Obviously, I was keeping all options open. It was the early eighties, and Larry Bird and company had just won one of their world championships. I was about eight or nine years old and really meant what I had written. I didn't think of myself as a trailblazer; I was at an age when I knew no gender. I was at an age when I thought I could do anything I wanted, and what I wanted was to play sports. I was also at an age when the physical differences between boys and girls were not very significant. In the summer I was perfectly comfortable without a shirt on shooting baskets in our driveway with my brother. Our chests looked pretty much the same. (Thank God that is no longer the case, and God, my brother thanks you, too.) Certainly taller, and probably stronger, than any of the boys in my class, I did not have any reason to think these circumstances would change. I also still believed in Santa Claus.

Now I'm a few years older and wiser. I've realized that I simply cannot play on a men's professional basketball team, but it wasn't easy to convince me of this.

I first saw the physical differences between the men's and women's games "up close and personal" the spring of my sophomore year in college. I was sitting in Gampel Pavilion after a shooting workout and our men's team was about to play pickup. They had only nine people and asked me if I'd like to join them. I ran to get my ankles taped and returned ready for action. The first time I got the ball on offense I was about four feet from the basket and took a hook shot that basically would have been unblockable in the women's game. A second after it left my hand I saw it fly in the opposite direction as Rudy Johnson leaped in the air and rejected it. After we ran down the court and got ready to play defense, I got position in the lane. Then I saw Donny Marshall drive past me with the basketball. I was not about to get in the way of this 225-pound guy.

My next time down the court my nose was broken. As one of my teammates went for a layup, I got on the other side of the hoop, in position to get the rebound in case he missed. I never expected him to hang in the air long enough to come over to my side of the basket before shooting. Upon landing, his shoulder went straight into my nose. It started bleeding immediately and I ran to the training room. I didn't start crying until I looked into the mirror and saw a nose shaped like the letter S on my face. (It was the first of many broken noses for me.) I begged the school doctor to make my nose straight again. He understood my concern; he didn't want me to spend the rest of my life tilting my head in the same direction I wanted to kiss. He thought that a young woman needed to keep her choices open.

In the third grade I thought I could compete with the men on that level. Now I realize that I can't, although one men's pro basketball team drafted me at the end of my senior year at UConn. It was flattering, but I knew it was just a publicity stunt.

Growing up, I was definitely a tomboy. I liked playing sports and doing anything active. That same year I wrote to President Reagan, I was the only girl who sat with the boys at lunch. Our classroom was assigned two long tables in the cafeteria, and I always chose to sit with the boys. After all, they were the ones I played games with at recess and sat with during classes. At that time, there were soccer and football for boys but nothing for girls to do, so, along with a few boys, I organized races and kickball. The girls were more into hanging around the jungle gym and talking. I never imagined there was anything peculiar about being friends with the guys; I never even gave it a second thought. But one day my teacher called me to her desk. I thought she was going to give me my grades just like she did with everyone else in the class. She gave me more than that.

It was clear from the start of the year, I think, that she didn't like me. Earlier that year, in front of the whole class she had accused me of cheating on a test. I had gone home and complained to my mother. Since it was the beginning of the year, she didn't want me to get off to a bad start. So she called and left a message for the teacher at the school. The next day, this teacher called out my name and, again in front of the whole class, asked me why my mother had called. I told her I didn't know why. She then hauled me out into the hall and asked me again. I said that I guessed it was because she had accused me of cheating when I hadn't. Then she said that if I were going to go home and tell my mother everything that happened in her class, it was going to be a long year.

The day she called me to the front of the class, she said things to me that she didn't say to the others. After giving me my report card (I got very good grades), she proceeded to tell me that I was too much of a tomboy. She said that I should dress and act more like a girl. She asked me why I was the only girl who sat with the boys at lunch. She addressed my appearance and the way I behaved. She said I had to change. I put my head down and didn't answer or look at her.

I wasn't getting into any trouble (at least not too much) or slacking in school. I wasn't breaking any rules I knew about. But for a reason that totally angered and confused me at the time, my teacher was "concerned."

I went home and told my mother what this teacher had said to me. I'll never forget her response because it was even more shocking than my teacher's comments. As I had stood in front of the teacher listening to her, I knew my mother well enough to know that I could count on her to back me up. I knew she would tell me it was perfectly fine to dress like a boy, but I never expected the intensity of her response. Mom became furious. She found my father and repeated the story to him. She kept saying how she could not *believe* the *nerve* of my teacher. My mother was so angry that I wished I hadn't told her. I was afraid she would say something to my teacher and, remembering the teacher's threat, that I would get into even more trouble. Kids are totally powerless in those kinds of situations. Adults sometimes forget this but I don't think I ever will.

If I were to get a letter now from a young girl describing a similar kind of prejudice, I would go to her school and tell that girl's teacher that she (or he) was wrong. It is impossible to expect a young boy or girl to stand up for him- or herself, particularly in front of friends and classmates. It is equally impossible to expect that you can legislate a change in others' attitudes. The only thing that can make a difference is the support of parents, school principals, and community leaders. Nobody else can protect a kid's sense of self.

Back then, I had yet to give much thought about what it meant to be a girl as opposed to a boy. (In fact, it wasn't until I got to high school that the whole issue of femininity came up. And even then, questions about it seemed centered on what kind of hairstyle I chose or what kind of makeup I might wear.) My mother raised her children to believe they could be anything they wanted. Now she had to deal with a teacher who was sending a very different message. Good thing my mom's message sounded louder and clearer in my head than this teacher's. If I had listened to the wrong woman, I would probably have thought there was something wrong or unfeminine about playing basketball. I would have thought there was something wrong with having friends who were boys. Luckily, my mom taught me well. I knew that there was nothing wrong with who I was.

I didn't change much after that lecture from my teacher. At the same time, I made sure I was no longer the only girl sitting with the boys at lunch, as I had arranged to have a couple of my girl friends join me at the boys' table. I didn't stop talking to the boys in class. If anything, I talked to them more. Just seeing my mother's response to what my teacher said hammered home to me that I was not to listen to that teacher. My teacher was right to say that one person in the class had to change. That one person was not the student. That one person was the teacher. I hope she sees now what I have made of myself. I hope she realizes that it was my difference from the girl she wanted me to become that got me where I am today.

As a ten-year-old, I can't imagine what I had to say to President Reagan. Like the rules of where to sit, how to dress, and who to talk to, the idea of the president of the United States seemed to have nothing to do with me, particularly since I wasn't as interested in becoming president as I was in playing ball for the Celtics. I'm beginning to understand, however, that our country's leaders have a lot to do with who we are and who we can become. A good president, I suppose, can be a lot like a good teacher, a good principal, or a good coach.

I'm forced to think about such things on a flight to Washington to jog with President Clinton.

I missed our team's visit to the White House because I was in Europe with the USA National Team. Unbeknownst to me, ever since that visit UConn alumni in Washington had been working with Connecticut's senators and representatives, trying to set up a time for me to meet the president. They had been touching base with my brother, Jason, but he didn't tell me exactly what they were up to. It was hard because all the planning took place right after I returned from Europe with the

National Team when I felt like there were a million strings attached to my body and a million hands pulling them in all different directions. I voiced my frustrations to my brother about my schedule, and apparently he felt it was better if he didn't mention that another string was attached.

So, following two weeks of nonstop appearances in Connecticut and day trips to New York for various events, my brother informed me of the possibility of meeting the president. We were in Boston for yet another banquet and he casually asked me if I would like to go running with the president. I was so tired and worn out that I said no. Of course, I didn't think that the offer was in any way serious. Two days later, when he told me that we were leaving for Washington, I felt a bit lost and overwhelmed. It wouldn't be the first or the last time I felt that way.

I met Jason and his boss David at their office and we drove together to the airport. Since the season ended I had gotten quite accustomed to flying first class, so I could do nothing but laugh when we pulled up to the ValuJet terminal. The plane was late in arriving so the three of us chatted and joked while we waited. We were quite certain that we were the only people in the airport who were going to meet the president. If not, we knew that any others were on a different airline! Fortunately, my brother got the seat next to the woman who never stopped talking, and I was able to sleep the entire flight. We arrived at the UConn Alumni Club about half an hour late. It was a good opportunity to meet new people and say a lot of thank you's as they continually congratulated me on our team's success. The number of people's lives that were touched by our basketball team will never cease to amaze me. I eventually crawled into bed around midnight. While I was lying in bed it finally hit me that in seven short hours I would be lacing up my Reeboks for a run with the president. Good thing I was completely exhausted or there is no way I would have fallen asleep.

Jason, David, and I were picked up by Ted Haddad from the UConn Club and driven to the White House. Jason and David were also dressed in running attire hoping they'd be able to jump in on the jog. After we cleared security and the car passed the sniff test by the dogs, we drove up to the front door of the White House. We felt good about everything except the fact that Ted had a big bumper sticker on the back of his Cadillac that read "Bob Dole for President." I could just imagine President Clinton seeing the sticker and telling me to take a hike over to Mr. Dole's office and ask *him* if he wanted to go for a run. Fortunately, Ted scraped the sticker off right after we arrived.

We sat in a room and waited for further instructions. Two other people who were running with the president that morning waited with us. One was a woman who worked at the White House whose husband was in the military and about to be shipped off somewhere, and the other was an old friend of the president's from Arkansas. At about 7:30 A.M. I looked up and saw President Bill Clinton walk through the doorway. He was yawning and stretching his arms over his head like most people do right after waking up. He wore black sweat pants and a black tee shirt, and I was pleased to see the UConn women's basketball National Champions hat given to him by my team perched on his head. His face was very red, but he basically looked exactly like he did on television. I don't know why he wouldn't have. He was fairly tall, about 6'2", and much thinner in person than I had imagined. I stood and greeted him. He asked me when I was going to Oxford. Apparently the aides who remembered to give him the UConn hat forgot to tell him that the Rhodes people booted me from consideration back in November. He also commented on our season and the team's visit to the White House.

The three invited runners and Mr. Clinton got into his limousine and took a ten-minute ride to the site of our jog. He chatted with us the whole time. The more he spoke, the more comfortable I felt. He talked about getting to sleep late because he was waiting up for Chelsea to get home the night before. That struck me as funny because my dad always had the same difficulty sleeping when his kids were out. He couldn't slip into his comfortable snore until all his children were home. The president also voiced his frustration with the fact that he was no longer able to run in downtown D.C. now that a person had opened fire on the White House with an automatic weapon. (I made no comparison to my father on this point.) At last, we reached the park where we were to run.

When we got out of the car, I realized how many people were with us. There had been police cars and vans following the limo the whole time. I hadn't really noticed them before. I felt bad that our president needs this kind of security, although I must admit I never felt so safe preparing to go for a jog.

We started our run and Jason and David were able to join in. I ran behind the president for the first one and a half miles, with the fear of catching the president's legs and tripping him never far from my mind. That would have been great for my image—I would have gone from Rebecca Lobo: the basketball player from Connecticut, to Rebecca Lobo: the woman who had shown up in a "Bob Dole for President" car and tripped Mr. Clinton from behind.

Right before we reached the press, the president invited me to run beside him. I was on his right when we reached the horde of photographers and journalists shouting questions to him about some vote. He smiled and ignored their inquiries. When we were out of earshot he remarked, "I never answer their questions." I had to laugh. We continued to chat until we finished the three-mile jog. I was so caught up in our run that I never noticed the boats on the river or the agents with binoculars along the riverbank looking for anything suspicious. What I did notice were the people's faces as we ran by them. Some were completely amazed while others acted as if they saw the president every day. I appreciated the ones who were nonchalant. They realized that the president was a human being just like they were. Then again, perhaps they were just Republicans.

My brother and David joined us in the limousine for the ride back to the White House. The limo was a bit cramped since four of the six people in it were over six feet tall. It also smelled quite a bit worse than the rose garden we were to walk through as soon as we arrived at the president's home. I don't remember if the windows in the car were tinted, but they didn't need to be because we fogged them up so completely on the return trip. The gossip columnists would have had a field day if they had seen the president's limousine drive by with those windows.

When we arrived, the president gave us a personal tour of the Oval Office and his private office. He took great pride in many of the personal objects on his shelves and delighted in giving us detailed descriptions of them. After about forty-five minutes, the president, responding to the impatience of his aides, went to start the rest of his day. I had been somewhat wary of keeping him from his job but he seemed a little reluctant to go. Afterward, we took a tour of the rest of the White House and then began the journey home. I no longer felt as oppressed as I had earlier, nor did I feel the tug of those millions of strings in the same way after that. Instead, as I settled down in my seat of a puddle-jumper airline, I felt relaxed and happy. Looking around, Jason, David, and I smiled and shared the secret pleasure of the day. Jason craned his head over the back of his seat and remarked, "Not a bad twenty-four hours, huh Bec!?!"

When I wrote that letter to Ronald Reagan, I may not have imagined that I would one day run with the president of the United States. I may not have dreamed that I would get a personal tour of the White House. However, I was never told by my parents that I could NOT do any of these things. I was never told by my parents I could NOT play for the Boston Celtics or the New York Giants. If I had heard such words, then perhaps I would have listened to my teacher, started having doubts about myself, my femininity, whatever. I never would have played basketball. I never would have run with the president. I never would have written a book.

When I look back, I see that growing up doesn't happen all at once or even gradually, but in fits and starts. The year I wrote to President Reagan, wrote the note about the substitute teacher's mustache, and was told to dress and act more like a lady, was also the year I stopped believing in Santa Claus. I came home from school one day and found my mother in the kitchen cooking dinner. I put my books down and asked her in a rush of words:

"Mom, the kids were talking at school and they said there was no Santa Claus. I said there was no Santa Claus, too, but then I remember that time when we didn't have a lot of money for Christmas, but we still got the Ping-Pong table. So people are telling me there is no Santa and I kind of think there is no Santa, but then things happen where I think there is one. So is there?"

My mom stopped stirring the pot on the stove and looked me straight in the eye and told me there was no such thing as Santa Claus. I started bawling and before I knew it she was crying, too. Just because she's my mom, I guess. When we finally stopped she said, "But, promise me not to tell Jason or your father because they don't know." I promised her.

Even without Santa and the Boston Celtics, I was taught that anything is possible. I wasn't born with that knowledge, I was *taught* it. Each day something happens in my life that proves it to be true.

★ RUTHANN

In the early years of my father's construction business, my mother worked at my dad's side digging ditches with a pick and shovel. Having worked at a gas station during the war, she thought nothing of poking around under the hood of a car or tackling a broken bicycle. When I wondered out loud what I would be when I grew up, she responded, "You can be whatever you want to be," and this was the legacy I passed on to my children.

It would be untrue to say that neither my mother nor I ever sent messages loaded with sexism of one kind or another. No one is immune to the subtle attitudes that etch their mark on our self-image, day in and day out. Interwoven with the words "You can be whatever you want to be" were the words "Act like a lady," and "Nice girls don't do that." So, as a parent, I was more appalled when I caught the girls spitting than I was when I caught Jason doing the same. I preferred shopping for jumpers over shopping for jeans. Sensing my bias, I heeded my own internal voice of reason and made a conscious effort to encourage the kids to chart their own course.

Remembering the fun my brother and I had playing with toy trucks and bulldozers in imitation of my father's business, I had no difficulty with the girls joining their brother in play with Matchbox cars and G. I. Joes. Barbie dolls were not allowed in our house. For some reason I had no problem with G. I. Joe's career choice, whereas the idea of Barbie left me cold. She was nothing but fluff. The Christmas and birthday gift requests of the three children frequently mirrored each other: three-car racing tracks with command control, an Evel Knievel doll and motorcycle, remote control cars, and locomotives with yards of track. The year Rachel and Rebecca received football uniforms for Christmas, they begged to wear them to the family gathering at their Aunt Pam's and Uncle Mark's. My immediate reaction was one of horror, for everyone would be all dressed up. Surely the girls would look out of place in football uniforms. I had to ask myself an important question: "Does it really matter?" So, off we went, football uniforms and all, to celebrate the holiday season.

I clearly remember the first time I confronted the actual opportunities for girls in the world of sports. It came as a jolt. Eight-year-old Rebecca announced proudly that she was going to play for the New York Giants when she grew up. I suddenly felt like a fraud. "I have always told Rebecca she could be whatever she wanted," I said to Dennis, "but the reality is she can't." I had fostered a belief in my child that was untrue, and I was angry. When Rebecca discovered that my mother had seats at the Boston Garden, near Red Auerbach, the general manager of the Boston Celtics at the time, she passed on a note to him saying she planned on being the first female player for the Celtics. How does a parent explain to a child that by virtue of his or her gender certain opportunities are unattainable? How could I explain to Rebecca that based not on her talents but on her sex she was an unlikely Boston Celtics star? It didn't make any sense. As Rebecca's interest and ability in sports increased, so too did my awareness of the limited opportunity available to women in athletics.

We were fortunate that Southwick's Recreation Center, a nonprofit volunteer organization, provided a number of athletic activities for both girls and boys in our community. Everyone was assigned to a team and everyone played. For years Rebecca sported a green baseball cap with a white A on the front. Den referred to her as "the hat with a kid under it." When she was ten, Rebecca registered for the newly organized girls' basketball team. We waited for practice schedules to be announced, and when none was forthcoming, I inquired about the delay. I was told that due to a lack of interest, no girls' program was underway. "Well," I stated, "if she can't play on a girls' team, she'll play on the boys' team." And so it was that she not only played on the boys' team, she earned a starting spot on the traveling team as well.

Unfortunately, as a young girl I was a genetic throwback when it came to sports. With the exception of high school basketball, I had little understanding, interest, or skill in athletics during my youth. All arms and legs, I was self-conscious about my lack of coordination and the way I looked in my blue gym bloomers. I was embarrassed to be seen with field hockey equipment dangling from my body. My mother encouraged me to try my hand anyway, but I lacked her athletic prowess. Although I did not inherit her innate talent to throw a football, I did absorb her unspoken message that it was okay for a female to discover the pleasure that comes from throwing a perfect pass.

Growing up during the fifties and sixties, I was keenly aware that the measure of a girl was more often her appearance than her mind or her athletic ability. Role models of the day were gleaned not from the academic or athletic arenas but from movie and fashion magazines. The round, full-figured look of Marilyn Monroe or Sophia Loren was the ideal to which young girls aspired. Much attention was focused on the female bustline, and I cringed in horror as a seventh grade classmate turned to me in homeroom, stared at my chest, and loudly interrogated, "RuthAnn, when are you going to bloom?" I remember diligently doing exercises that promised a bigger bust measurement. I also remember spending an inordinate amount of time sitting in front of the mirror applying facials, makeup, and nail polish. I tortured my hair into shape with a teasing comb. I worried about the size of my nose and begged my mother for a nose job. When Dennis asked me to marry him years later without ever mentioning my nose, I realized that the most important thing about my nose was that it worked!

At 5′11″ I was exceptionally tall in comparison to my peers. Surrounded by friends and family who seldom did more than call me a "long drink of water" or "Long Tall Sally," I was rarely conscious of my height except when asked to dance by a shorter boy. I remember the look of astonishment on the face of a young man when I stood up to accept his invitation—he only came up to my chest! Behind him, his friends sniggered. I asked him, "It doesn't bother me, does it bother you?" He shook his head no and, to the astonishment of his friends, we enjoyed each other's company for the remainder of the dance.

Finding clothes that fit was another matter. Too often I had to buy a larger size in order to get a longer hemline. Unlike the baggy look so popular today, the fitted look was in during my teen years but my clothes were usually a size or two bigger. Salespeople would tug at my sleeve and try to convince me that a cuff above my wrist was a fashionable "bracelet length." I was told that the solution to wearing shorter sleeves was to push them up. I suspect that I prefer the longer look today because it was impossible to find years ago. And when a salesperson suggests that either my daughters or I push up our sleeves, I go into quiet spasm and quickly put the article back on the rack. Shoes were an even bigger problem. It seemed my foot was always one size bigger than the largest size in the store. I had little choice in style and often ended up cramming my toes into pointy shoes that didn't fit.

Like all girls my age, I wanted to be pretty. My mother, raised in a large working-class family, wanted me not only to be pretty but to be educated and socially polished. She would not have me cleaning houses, working as a cook, and digging ditches as she had. During my junior year of high school, she enrolled me in a six-week course at the John Robert Powers School in Boston. There I learned makeup application, how to enter a car without showing my behind, and how to tackle a complicated table setting. Although I take pleasure in knowing which spoon to use when, I have since learned to distinguish between civility and surface charm. I have recognized that good grooming can be a mark of self-respect rather than a tool for female vanity.

Remembering my mother's help during my own unsteady approach to womanhood, I offered the Powers course to my daughters. Neither was interested. Maybe we have to find new ways to see our daughters safely through this passage. I want to believe that messages about the importance of talent over looks are different for young girls today, but the covers of teen magazines and conversations with girls tell me otherwise. Articles abound not only on personal appearance but on how to enhance one's sex appeal. What can we be thinking?

My personal observations support the research that finds that these messages cause adolescent girls to lose their self-esteem, shut down in class, and measure themselves not by their accomplishments but in the reflections of their boyfriends' eyes. I have seen young girls develop eating disorders after being teased about their eating habits. I have heard mothers worry because their daughters are not as popular as others. At a recent parade I spotted a little girl no older than five sporting a sash with "Little Miss Something" on it. I was horrified to think that at her young age this little girl was already being taught to value herself in terms of her looks. And although my daughters were disinterested in the finishing school, they nevertheless primped in front of the mirror for hours upon hours. I remember Dennis telling Rachel as she perused the class superlatives in a school yearbook that being voted best looking is a curse one has to live with for the rest of his or her life. I often reminded my children that looks fade with time; effort is better put toward developing one's gifts and talents.

When I reflect on my past, I realize that although I witnessed independence in my mother and was encouraged by her to keep my sights high, I also heard the quiet whispers of a society at large. My school counselor never talked to me about careers outside of teaching and nursing. Even Mom encouraged the field of education because she thought it complemented the role of homemaker and mother. I remember childhood friends like Edna who dreamed of veterinary school; it was beyond her reach. My high school had restricted some classes by gender; when I inquired about the woodworking class, I was told it was "for boys only." Home economics was "for girls."

Unlike many schools at the time, we were fortunate to have athletic programs for girls. Nevertheless, those of us who played basketball did so by an archaic set of rules and were limited to half-court play and two dribbles. Athletic scholarships for girls were never mentioned; they didn't exist. When we took Rebecca to see *A League of Their Own*, I was touched by the hardships and humiliation those women endured in order to play a game they loved. I lectured as we left the theater, "I hope young women today appreciate those who have gone before them. You're playing ball today because others before you were willing to make sacrifices. Don't take it for granted."

My hope for girls today lies in the adults who surround them. I have noticed that the fathers of girls are sometimes more in tune than their mothers in wanting equal opportunities for their daughters. One mother told me that her husband, an avid sports fan, became a feminist the moment their daughter was born. Yet maybe if this man had had a boy first, his daughter wouldn't have gotten his attention in the same way. Men are beginning to discover that the kind of relationship they had reserved for their future sons can be found with their daughters. Den taught both my daughters how to throw a softball properly, using their entire body instead of just their arm. He helped them soup up their bicycles; he bought them skateboards. Den's involvement in their lives wasn't always just a matter of his athletic interests either. He was, for example, great at keeping current with popular music. This is as sure a way as any to have something to talk about with a teenager. The key isn't what you are talking about or doing together but in finding common interests and activities, engaging them in conversations that go beyond "What did you learn in school today."

At conferences, I continually remind female teachers that the young women in their classrooms are watching them closely. It is imperative that they not tolerate crude comments in the classroom or the faculty lounge. In my first job teaching at a state school for troubled children, as one of two females on the staff, I was relegated to the coffee detail. I wouldn't do that today. If teachers respond to discrimination and harassment according to the law, their students will learn how to handle similar situations in the world they'll face outside the classroom. Mothers should do the same. It isn't enough to give lip service, to tell daughters that they can do anything; women need to support girls' athletic events and scholarship drives. If I look in the paper and I see a woman advertising her plumbing skills, I'll give her a shot first. Women need to become politically active and aware when women's issues are being debated in Congress. By women's issues I mean health care issues, child care issues, equal opportunity issues.

We need to cry "Foul" when Madison Avenue manipulates and demeans our image for commercial purposes. Although I am still smarting from the feminist rhetoric of the sixties, I do acknowledge that, thanks to those ladies, my awareness of the ways in which women are used to sell things and to fatten pocketbooks is much sharper now than it was when I was a young woman. The truth of it is that if they hadn't been out there thumping the drums, I would probably still be watching June Cleaver vacuuming in her skirt and pearls. I do believe in equality for human beings, and I am willing, now, to do battle to make it happen.

As luck would have it, I was asked to act as the Title IX compliance coordinator for the Granby school district in the late 1980s, a role I continue to share today with a colleague, Barbara

Cohen. Title IX specifically prohibits sexual harassment and gender discrimination in schools accepting public monies. Workshops and conferences exposing the gender-based inequities in our society have heightened my sensitivity to the injustices perpetrated on our young people, and I've since recognized that whenever we limit any individual from developing his or her talents, we all lose in the process.

Barbara and I have been working diligently—through classroom lessons, parent and staff workshops, and conference presentations—to raise the level of awareness of gender discrimination among students, parents, and educators. I often meet women who respond to this subject with the same objections I once had. "This whole thing has just gone too far. You are out to unisex everyone. Men and women *are* different." (If you haven't looked lately, men and women are different. But we have more in common than our body parts might suggest.) There are men whose jaws begin working, who tense up and defend themselves: "I don't discriminate in my class and I never have discriminated. I treat everybody the same." I guarantee you these men are the biggest sexists going. Then there are those men who are sensitive, who agonize, who take what we are trying to say to heart but who, at the same time, are bewildered. They feel accused of something they don't understand. "I'm afraid to do or say anything in my class for fear of being misinterpreted." I worry about these men who are truly our allies. We will lose their patience and support if we lapse into a "we versus them" debate.

The most frustrating people I have encountered are those who refuse to accept the idea of sexual discrimination. It is amazing how quickly these people sit up and pay attention when their own ox is gored, when they find out, like I did, that there is a boys' basketball team but not one for girls. This converts many to the idea, even proselytizers like myself. A little humble pie can go a long way.

Communities still exist where physical education classes are divided not by skill level but by sex. There are teachers who are still tempted to segregate students in this way for group work, spelling and math bees, or classroom chores. One wise gentleman suggested the following test when segregating kids: If you substitute a racial, religious, or ethnic category for "boys here," "girls there" and the result raises the hair on the back of your neck, then think again. I am convinced that most people who discriminate do so because of ignorance. We are products of a society that has differentiated gender roles for centuries; we are frequently unaware of our own limitations, denials, and fears that hinder young people from discovering their talents and pursuing their interests.

Sexual harassment is an equally disturbing aspect of discrimination. When workshop participants claim they have few or no complaints in their school districts, I know they have failed to get the word out to their students and staff; people don't report if they are unaware of what to report or to whom. Victims of harassment too often think they are powerless to affect change or, worse still, they think that they are responsible for initiating the harasser's behavior. The impact on a student can be devastating.

A friend of mine confided that her high school son had been the unwelcome recipient of a female teacher's affection. When her son, embarrassed and confused by his teacher's behavior, reported the incident to school authorities, he was asked if he had encouraged her. A definite no-no! The teacher was responsible for her actions, yet she was allowed to resign without consequence, thus sending a subtle message to the student that the needs of the teacher were more important than his. Left to fend for himself, he wrestled for years with the emotional turmoil resulting from the school's irresponsible action.

At one of our workshops, a mother relayed how her fifth-grade daughter was being taunted by a boy in her class. He wrote her notes of a sexual nature, leered at her across the classroom, and joked about her with his friends. She stopped participating in classroom activities. She became withdrawn and cried easily. She dreaded going to school. It wasn't until her mother attended one of our workshops and subsequently talked with her teacher that action was taken: After confronting the perpetrator and talking with his parents, the principal of the school changed the boy's classroom in addition to offering counseling. The girl in turn was assured that her rights had been violated, that she was not to blame, and that her rights were protected by law. Within weeks she had resumed her bubbly nature and again began volunteering in class.

It is not uncommon for students testing the waters of adolescence to find themselves floating dangerously close to the riptide of harassment. Facing an onslaught of hormonal confusion, lacking dating experience, and spurred on by mass marketing and media, they blunder forward by trial and error in their encounters with the opposite sex with little more than MTV as their guide. I am amazed by the number of kids who fashion their concepts of relationships after soap operas or television sitcoms. Pretty frightening! Den and I recently removed a movie channel from our home after finding explicit sex scenes on at 9:00 P.M. "My children are grown," I reported to the cable company, "but I teach middle-school students. I am not going to support this kind of garbage for those kids to see."

I don't consider myself a prude nor am I put off by sexual innuendos, but I am offended when marketers think innuendos are the only means to attract and hold attention. I am equally offended by their lack of concern for the impact their messages have on kids. I am tired of combating the language and behavior kids adopt from television, movie, and music video personalities. I am sick of the sexually explicit drawings and the four-letter words that have replaced the occasional "Damn" once scribbled on bathroom walls. To those who argue that educators must teach kids how to handle what they see and hear today, I counter that kids are not yet ready; it is akin to asking a four-year-old to understand the intricacies of algebra.

It's too bad that I wasn't more Title IX savvy when Rebecca was told by her teacher to dress like a girl. Title IX is more than a mandate for dealing with glaringly discriminatory or harrassing behavior, although that is what most people associate with the law. The day-to-day subtle insinuations can be even more harmful to a child's emotional well-being. I have to believe this teacher knew what she was doing.

I want my daughters to enjoy being women, but never at the cost of being themselves. Who knows, perhaps the next president of the United States to be found jogging along the Potomac will be a former tomboy.

★ 4 ★

Family Is as Family Does

★ *REBECCA*

The summer before my senior year at UConn, I worked in a basketball camp and met a sixth grader named Lauren. I became her coach. She was a good kid—hard working and honest—with a great sense of humor; I could see a little of myself in her. The day she left, she gave me a pair of earrings that I still wear practically nonstop. We both had tears in our eyes when it came time to say good-bye.

We stayed in touch after that. She'd call me up to tell me what was going on, how school was, how basketball was. She told me about the boys she liked and which boys liked her. Sometimes a friend of hers got on the line too and we'd have a three-way conversation. Often it's hard to find something to say to younger kids—she's about fourteen now—but she was more like a little sister to me. One day not too long ago she called me and said, "You're not going to believe this," and then she began telling me how she read about kids her age who were having contests to see who could have the most sex in one day! I didn't believe it but she insisted it was true. I told her that if she ever told me she was having sex too, I would come down right then and there and give her a whupping! "You better *never*," I said.

When I was growing up I often thought it might be nice to have a younger sister or brother. I dreamed about looking after them in the same way my brother always looked after me. Now I'm glad I don't have a younger sister, because if she played basketball, for instance, people would constantly compare her to me. With Lauren, I care about what happens to her, and I want to keep my eyes open. If she ever needed anything she could get it from me. Luckily, she also has parents she can rely on, but I think it's easier for her to have someone like me to talk to because she doesn't think of me as a real adult. I thought of my brother Jason the same way.

When I was in grade school and middle school my brother could do no wrong. I watched his every move. He was known to his high school basketball teammates as the "Gentle Giant." Sitting on the bleachers behind his team's benches, I would prop my chin on my hands and eavesdrop on every word that passed between the coach and his team. If Jason missed his shots or the team lost, I parroted the coach's criticisms on the ride home. Eight years old to his fourteen, eleven years old to his seventeen, we could never really have a relationship like that of good friends. He either picked on me or parented me. I took everything he said to heart, particularly his scoldings but also his encouragement. I valued his words almost as much as my parents'.

People were always talking about what a great guy Jason was, noting that he always knew what to say and was unfailingly unselfish when it came to giving credit to his teammates. He didn't care if a person was popular or unpopular, he treated everyone equally well. As a child I heard this talk and wanted more than anything to have people say the same things about me. And, if possible, I wanted them to say even better things about me. Jason was everything I thought an athlete should be, but I wasn't above competing with him. The first time I beat him at Horse, the whole neighborhood heard about it.

Jason wasn't just that way at school or playing sports. At home, he paid a lot of attention to Rachel and me. At night, he helped us to imagine spiders crawling underneath our beds. At bathtime he collected handfuls of carpet fuzzies to drop in our bathwater. He once helped us bury eighteen old juice cans in the yard so we could have our own miniature golf course. After a couple of weeks and a few rainstorms, our golf course doubled as a mosquito farm. He directed the construction of forts in the upstairs hallways, organizing wars and assaults on each others' fortifications with balls made from old socks. He refereed our boxing matches, waiting impatiently for one of us to hit the other too hard with down mittens. When that happened and the bawling began, Jason always convinced us that Mom and Dad weren't really interested in how Rachel got a bloody nose. "It's just too boring," he would say. He really enjoyed figuring out just how much torture he could get away with. We adored him.

In high school, when he went off to play football with his buddies, he'd always let Rachel and me tag along, even though we were the only girls and were so much younger. After much begging, he let us join the neighborhood Nerf ball games. I know it must have been a nuisance, but he never said a word. Even when he went away to college, after his weekend games he'd come back to the motel to spend time with us when I know there was probably a party he would rather have gone to.

Now that I am twenty-two and my brother is twenty-eight, things have changed a lot between us. Each year I was in college the gap closed more and more. Now we talk about almost everything. His fills me in on his career and his love life. "Tell your baby sister all about it," I say to him. Then I fill him in on basketball, my ever-changing relationship with our parents, and my own love life. And when, not too long ago, he tried to give me some pointers on my shots in the family driveway, I turned to Rachel (who was a player in two NCAA tournaments and an assistant coach in two more) and said, "Gee Rachel, what do you think? I've played in an NCAA tournament, you've played in an NCAA tournament. Excuse me, Jason, where did you say you had played?" Now he has begun referring to the fact that he had higher SAT scores. I don't feel like his "little sister" anymore, and he no longer thinks of me that way, either, even though that's what I'll always be.

My relationship with Rachel is completely different from my relationship with Jason. She is only two and a half years older, but people often assumed I was the older sister because I was taller. When we were younger, we did everything together, competing against each other and against ourselves. She pitched, I batted. I pitched, she batted. We played Horse or One on One; we raced bicycles or had swimming contests. In high school, things changed. Rachel became the black sheep of the family. She is the only kid out of the three of us who ever tried to run away and was the child who got in the most trouble. She never really liked studying and would put it off until way past bedtime. She also always enjoyed testing my parents' rules on curfew and everything else. Out way past curfew one night with friends, she had my mother calling all the area hospitals and police stations. Then again, my mother does tend to overreact in certain situations. But my sister was always the best at getting my mother to do it.

I was in middle school when we started to argue a lot, mostly about stupid things like borrowing each other's clothes or who controlled the remote to the TV. Maybe we missed Jason's refereeing skills. There was a time when Rachel considered me a prude and a goody two shoes. She thought I judged her; she was right. One time when she was a freshman or sophomore in high school, she came home and told me that she had had a beer. My reaction was, "What, you think you're *cool*, now?" After that she thought of me as a little sister, rather than the person she used to play Wiffle ball with in the back yard. She knew I wouldn't tell Mom or anything; she just didn't want me to be her walking conscience. I missed her after that.

By the time I got to high school, she was more involved with her friends than I was with mine, and she went to parties more often than I did. And, inevitably perhaps, she had a boyfriend and I didn't. I still preferred to do the things she and I had done together when we were younger, but stopped asking her to join me. We were on the same high school basketball team, and though we both had big hair and very long legs, there were big differences too. Her jersey number was 13 and mine was 31. That about describes our relationship back then.

Traveling to Dartmouth on weekends to watch Jason play basketball brought the family back together in a way. We stayed in a motel with my parents in one double bed and Rachel and me in the other. The rooms were not very big, but there was plenty of space. The only time we got in each other's way was when everyone wanted a piece of the mirror in the morning. We drove my dad crazy as each woman took her turn shellacking her hair with spray. The fumes in the air gave him a great excuse to go to the lobby and get coffee. He always returned with a cup for himself and a cup for my mom. If I were lucky, the hotel also had hot chocolate and if they did, guaranteed my dad returned with a cup for me. Even now, hot chocolate reminds me of those mornings.

As Rachel was around less and less, I began to keep a journal. I had had a diary when I was in elementary school (Rachel got a diary first and so I had to have one, too). I kept mine hidden behind some books on a shelf in my room, so naturally I forgot about it for long stretches of time. I don't think I filled it up until I was almost in high school. When I got a journal, I moved my hiding place to under my mattress. I'm sure my mom saw it but she never read it because that's the way she is.

After Rachel went away to college, things changed again. She came home most weekends to visit her boyfriend, and we sat on our beds and talked just like we used to. By the time I got to college, we were very close. Now we talk on the phone every day (don't you love it when people have an 800 number at work?) and tell each other everything that's going on. There are things I know about her that no one else does and vice versa. Although I doubt she ever read my journal, she'd never need to because I tell her everything anyway. Of course, we can't fight over clothes anymore because we wear such different sizes, and we each have our own TVs and our own remotes. We now talk about how hard it is not to let yourself be defined by how you look or how tall you are. I think she'll do some great things in life. She's no longer the black sheep—except in summer when she gets a tan we all envy. She's a beautiful person with a heart of gold. She's no longer just a friend, she's my best friend. I'm not sure how it happened, but I know we'll be close for the rest of our lives.

Now, too, Rachel and I see eye-to-eye on most things. Like me, she craves our parents' approval, which is probably why it was so difficult for her when she was younger. We all strive to please them, to not let them down. If Rachel handed them her report card and it didn't have straight As on it, she'd feel awful. My parents always tried to treat us fairly; they didn't judge us on how many points we scored or how good our grades were compared to our siblings'. But when you're younger, it's easy to confuse parental expectations with the terms of approval and love.

I suppose everyone wants parental approval. I always cared what my parents thought, about everything. Even when I told them I was going to do something whether they liked it or not, in my heart I wanted them to like it. When I was at odds with my parents or very angry with them, I looked to my brother or sister to help me figure out where exactly *they* were wrong.

Most of the time, of course, I agreed with my parents' values. When I answer letters from fans who are having trouble with something and asking for advice, I can certainly recommend general principles. "Be a good person and study hard," I urge.

"Don't do drugs," I'll tell someone else. "Treat other people, no matter who they are, with respect and dignity and fairness."

People live by different values and standards. Maybe this person did something bad, but you have no idea what his or her background is or what circumstances may have led up to it. I'm always willing to listen to people; usually they need that more than anything. When it comes to advice, I'm much happier giving pointers on basketball. Although I wasn't always this way, when it comes to judging people or being critical of them, I'm now reluctant. Perhaps I learned from my experience with Rachel.

The one time my mother and I profoundly disagreed on something occurred the summer that I worked in the tobacco fields. I was fourteen years old.

Working in the tobacco fields was hard work. The first part of the summer we spent outside tying up the tobacco plants whose leaves were later used to wrap cigars. It was particularly hard when the plants were small and I had to lean all the way down to the plant. First I pulled a string from a bucket on my back and tied the end to the top of the plant, making a special knot. Then I stood up and tied the other end to a wire above the plant. We taped our hands everyday so that we could break off the string after we tied it to the wire. Then on to the next plant, lean over, tie knot, stand up, tie knot, break the string, step over, lean down—for eight hours. I could get going fairly fast but it was really painful on my hamstrings, and my hands got all cut from breaking the strings. The string trained the plant to grow straight, and as the plant got taller we had to wrap more string around the leaves and wind it about the stalk to keep it growing straight. (Just like raising kids, I suppose.) Once the plants reached the right height, they were moved into huge, hot, dark barns where the leaves were sewn and packed for shipment. There were piles and piles of leaves and each leaf had to be lifted up to a machine up above. Because each machine was the same height, every morning I went in I had to dig a foot-deep hole in the dirt floor to stand in or else I'd be bending over all day.

It was miserable. I went home dirty, tired, and sore. But there was a consolation. Also working there was a guy named Rob who happened to be nineteen years old, just out of his freshman year of college. At the beginning of the summer he was interested in my sister but that never came to anything. As the summer went on, Rob and I became good friends. He had a quick wit and we'd bust on each other all day. He said he didn't know many people who could bust him back the way I did. One night he asked me to the movies and I enthusiastically said yes. I was so used to having guys for friends, I didn't think of it as a date. He probably thought of it as taking his little sister out to the movies. When I went home, I asked my mom if I could go and she said I could. Looking back, I think I may have led her to believe that a few more people would be going with us, however, I didn't feel as if I was lying. Besides, I trusted Rob.

We went to the movies and grabbed an ice cream on the way home. He got me back to the house before ten o'clock. My only thought as the car pulled up in front of our house was that I had to get inside before my father saw us because there were just the two of us in the car; Rob didn't even have time to park before I darted out the door. When I got up to my room I said to myself, "Oh my gosh, what if that was a date? I wonder if he might have kissed me if I hadn't run out of the car so fast, *what was I thinking*? I didn't even give him a *chance* to like me that way." I guess I was pretty innocent.

We went out about a week later with a group of friends. On the way home Rob asked if I wanted to go to the beach with him and another friend from work the next day. By then I was really excited. This was the first guy who had really shown an interest in me. He was the first boy I felt comfortable bringing home to meet my mom. And he could look past the braces and big hair and see me for who I was. When I was dropped off, I ran into the house and asked my mother if I could go to the beach. At first she said no, but after persistent begging she said she'd give me a firm answer in the morning.

The next morning I went down to breakfast wearing my bathing suit underneath my clothes. When I reached the bottom of the stairs, my father came up and asked, "What do you want in your lunch?" Of course I started crying right away.

"I'm not going to work," I said, "I'm going to the beach."

"No you're not."

"You said I could."

"Well, talk with your mother." So I did what any mature fourteen-year-old would do. I ran upstairs crying and screaming at my mother.

"I *am* going to the beach."

"No, you're not."

"Why not?"

"Because you have to go to work."

And so on and so forth. She wouldn't relent. All night I had been so happy about going. I thought for sure they would let me go, but instead I heard, "Your father and I decided that you are not going."

I only lasted until noon at work that day. I could not bear to sew tobacco leaves in a dark, smelly barn while my thoughts were of sunny, sandy beaches. I got a ride home and continued my pouting. After being home only fifteen minutes, my mom and dad suggested we go to a matinee of *Die Hard*. Since I was in love with Bruce Willis at the time, I couldn't say no. I quickly forgot the promise I made that morning to never forgive my mother and enjoyed the movie thoroughly. I didn't bring home another boy for six years.

I still think that my mom should have let me go to the beach. She still thinks she made the right decision. I thought she was doubting my ability to select friends and doubting my judgment of people. She thinks he was too old and I was too young. We still debate this point today. Of course, now that I'm older and have seen what college guys can be like, I understand my mother's position a little bit better. However, Rob was a great guy. I think my judgment, even as a fourteen-year-old, was pretty good.

If it were a tug-of-war between me and my mother over the beach issue, we would still both be pulling. It's one issue that we probably will never agree on. As for Rob, we stayed in touch for a little while, but now I have no clue where he is or what he's doing. I must admit I sometimes wonder if he watched my team win the national championship or if he saw my picture in the paper. Who knows what the answer is.

I've read many times how steel becomes as strong as it is only after being hammered and pounded over and over again. I imagine that relationships between people work the same. However fiercely we argue, the bonds between my parents and myself and my mother and myself seem only to toughen. And when she was battling her cancer, the bonds between my brother and sister and me hardened. We shared the same fears and the same thoughts. No one knew our mother like we did. We felt first how her survival was crucial to *our* survival. While she was fighting her battle with cancer, we were fighting the mere notion of living without her. During the months of her chemotherapy, I talked to Jason and Rachel constantly on the phone. I saw them at games. Each time, our conversation would turn to how mom was doing physically and how each of us was doing mentally. We agreed how lost we'd be without her, how we would not know what to do.

Luckily, we have not had to learn how to live without our mother. Instead, we have learned how siblings can become best friends.

★ *RUTHANN*

One evening, a long time ago, Den and I took Jason, who was about three, to a potluck supper. Almost immediately, Jason went dashing off with Dennis following in hot pursuit. Some sort of scolding must have followed because a young man in his early twenties came up to us and chided, "You want to watch your son grow up over the years, you don't want to help him grow up." It was such an odd comment that Den and I often reflected on it. As our children encountered the challenges of reaching adulthood, we were more likely to help rather than watch.

There is, of course, a fine line between helping and interfering, and as the kids grew older it was difficult to recognize the difference. I tended to overprotect, sometimes to the point of absurdity. Jason once negotiated a fifteen-mile bike trek by avoiding the main highways to reach his destination. I made him tell me his exact route and call me immediately when he arrived there. He was fourteen years old! Imagine, then, how I felt when several years later ten-year-old Rebecca returned from school one day and announced that she had missed the bus that morning. "How did you get to school?" I asked. School was six miles away and a good portion of the distance was along a major interstate. "Why, I rode my bike," she responded without blinking an eye. It occurred to me that perhaps I needed to give my kids a little more freedom than I was accustomed to as a child.

All the same, I took most of my lessons from my mother. While sitting around after my ten-year high school reunion, I listened to several high school friends relate the impact my mother had on their lives. One woman, who had grown up in an alcoholic home, thanked my mom for accepting her during childhood and modeling a stable home. Another woman echoed that tale and emphasized that ours was the only caring and welcoming home she knew. I was amazed. I recall feeling annoyed as a kid that my friends were often more interested in spending time with my mother than me; suddenly the picture cleared.

My mom was always involved in my activities. She labored over elaborate Halloween costumes that turned me into a sweet old-fashioned girl complete with bonnet and bustle. As my 4-H leader, she taught me how to cook and sew. As my Girl Scout leader, she marched me off into the woods, taught me how to make a trench fire and a bed roll, and revealed the mysteries of toasted marshmallows and s'mores. Den and I have tried to participate similarly in our children's lives. Our kids always had someone rooting for them while they were on the soccer, kickball, or softball fields or the basketball courts. Playing schedules sometimes found us running between fields as each of the three kids became involved in sports. Whether it was an elementary school production, a concert, a sports banquet, or a National Honor Society induction, at least one of us was there. The kids attended our events as well. They enjoyed watching Den coach and attended the conferring of my masters degree in psychology and counseling.

The greatest challenge in raising children is instilling discipline. I have often heard myself repeat the very words I heard as a child from my own parents. "Because I'm the mother, that's why," or "Because I said so!" Although Den and I gave our children the opportunity to voice their opinions, the final decisions were ours as heads of the house. We kept restrictions to a minimum, but we were firm in upholding the ones that we established. Each of us handled individual incidents as they occurred; we never believed in "Wait until Dad/Mom comes home." We also worked in tandem, not allowing the children to play one parent against the other.

In establishing rules for the kids, we again asked the all-important question, "Does it really matter?" Although we sometimes cringed at clothing or hairstyles that our kids wore to school, they were not issues we chose to argue over. During second or third grade, Rachel insisted on wearing one of two sweaters repeatedly to school. I was convinced that her teacher thought she only had those two items in her wardrobe. We did have to put our foot down, however, when wearing men's boxers became the in thing. To the girls' various arguments in defense of this style I responded, "You are not going to school in your father's underwear!" Nevertheless, Den became suspicious when, on a trip to the men's room, he discovered that someone had sewn the fly of his boxer shorts closed. When Rebecca and Rachel were in middle school, they graduated to "big hair" and turned a deaf ear to any subtle suggestions I offered. Today when they look in horror at high school pictures and ask me why I didn't say anything about their hairstyles, I respond in the same way my mom did when I asked the same question: "I tried to tell you but you wouldn't listen!"

We stressed the value of honesty, integrity, and loyalty to our children. As a first grader, Rachel had a longing for stickers. One day I found a stash of stickers in her lunchbox that I knew were not hers. Further investigation revealed that the stickers belonged to her teacher. The booty was returned and I remembered to add stickers to my Christmas shopping list. Rebecca's longing was for erasers. One afternoon she returned home from a neighbor's house with an eraser in hand.

"Where did you get that?" I asked.

"From Julie's house," she replied.

"Does she know you have it?" I persisted.

It was evident by the look on her face that she had helped herself to the eraser. I turned her toward the door and watched from the window with an aching heart as my four-year-old hesitatingly measured her steps to Julie's house to "fess up."

We often encouraged our children to test their talents and interests, helping them to establish priorities at the same time. Throughout his thirty years of coaching a number of sports, my husband has noted a change in the attitude and dedication of athletes. In an effort to "do it all," students frequently make appointments or schedule vacations at the expense of their training or the team's success. Once our kids made a commitment to a team or an organization, we expected them to honor it. Vacations during school breaks were unheard of when they came in the middle of a sporting season. One year Rebecca begged for tap dancing lessons. I dutifully took her to the studio where she mastered her shuffle, hop, step, with gangly arms and legs in motion. Six weeks prior to the dance recital, she announced that she wanted to quit. I firmly explained that she had made a commitment to her teacher and her class and she would be allowed to quit only after she had fulfilled that commitment. In a sequined costume and with one lone feather in her hair, she did her thing on stage with grim determination, then put aside her tap shoes forever.

On another occasion, Rachel, an exceptional musician, signed up to try out for a youth orchestra in nearby Springfield, Massachusetts. As the time approached for her tryout, she became extremely apprehensive and nervous. Tears began to flow as we headed off in the car. I could feel my frustration level rising. Finally I looked at her and reasoned, "This simply isn't worth all of this anguish. If you really want to turn around and go home we will. But first, tell me what's the worst that can possibly happen?" She sniffled, "I won't be selected." "That's right," I continued. "And the best that can happen is that you will make it. But if we turn around now you will never know." She chose to audition and was selected to perform with the orchestra.

As the parents in the house, Den and I monitored curfews and bedtime. Accustomed to a midnight curfew right up until my wedding day, I found it hard to adjust to the desires of a new generation, which comes alive at ten o'clock at night. Our kids were not allowed to go out on a school night unless it was for a school event, and weekend curfews were adjusted according to age and event but never extended beyond midnight. And anyone who was out of the house, including Den and myself, had to leave a number where he or she could be reached in case an emergency arose at home. Rachel tested our curfew on one occasion when she called from a local pizza parlor to inform us that "the crowd" was staying out and her ride would bring her home a little later. Den hopped in the car and went to pick her up.

"Only drink soda," I casually reminded Jason as he left to attend a party celebrating his team's entry into a tournament. It never occurred to me that he would do anything else, but he arrived home with beer on his breath. He explained that he and a friend had split a bottle of beer, which he held the rest of the evening.

"Listen, Jason," I countered, "nobody knows if that was your first or your tenth beer. People talk." Sure enough, when I arrived home the following Monday, I encountered my crestfallen son.

"Coach called me into his office. He heard I drank beer at the party. Kids that weren't even there are saying things that aren't true." Jason, who valued his reputation, was beside himself.

"Look, Jason," I responded, "you don't owe anyone an explanation except Coach and your teammates. But remember, you enjoy being well-thought-of and a role model. With that comes responsibility. There will always be someone happy to see you fall."

My biggest battle with Rebecca came when she wanted to go to the beach with several kids with whom she worked in the tobacco fields. It appeared to me that the kids were going in couples. She was only fourteen and the boy showing interest in her was nineteen. I flatly refused permission. I said she was too young and he was too old. She said he was only a friend. I wouldn't budge. Her anger and disappointment tumbled forth. She insisted I was old-fashioned and unreasonable. I snapped, "Keep it up and you'll be two inches shorter and a point guard!" To this day we debate the wisdom of my decision. There have been parental calls that I replay in my head and regret, but not this one.

When it came to sex, I wanted to give my children more than the cacophony of "Don'ts" my mother had bombarded me with from the onset of puberty until my walk down the aisle. (In Mom's defense, my sex education, however limited, was more extensive than hers had been. She learned the facts of life on her wedding night.) Like many women of my generation, I held at bay the passionate demands of the men I dated:

"I need a complete relationship."

"I desire you."

And once, to my horror, "My wife doesn't understand me."

Lifted from B movies and torrid romance novels, these were the clichés that I heard during those years. The more eloquently they pressed their case, the more I feared losing the relationship. Largely silent, our struggles in the front seat of a car were punctuated by my demure deflections:

"No."

"No!"

"No!"

This was the extent of my conversation on the topic of sex with any of my various boyfriends.

I, too, believe in Don'ts, but I also believe in an openness about sex that would be unimaginable to my mother. Today, young people need to learn a way to talk about their feelings that openly addresses both their emotional and physical longings. Popular culture cannot be relied upon to script these exchanges for them. If you can't talk truthfully about what's going on, I tell my students, you don't really know what *is* going on. Abstinence is not just about saying no, it is about giving oneself time to experience the upheaval and satisfactions of truly caring for another person.

On occasion, of course, I brought my sex education lesson plans home. My efforts to launch dinner table conversations about love, sexual responsibility, and the mortal dangers of sexually transmitted diseases went completely unappreciated but, I assume, not unheard. Hoping to test the limits of my candor, I suppose, the ever curious Rachel inquired one evening,

"How often do you and Daddy . . . you know?"

"Every Tuesday, without fail, Nosy Rosie."

As the kids grew older, we urged them to think critically about the kinds of messages pop culture bombarded them with—the lyrics, the commercials, the TV shows—and the value systems they represented. The ever present topic of to have or not to have premarital sex was the least fertile subject for lively family debate. I do not and will never approve of sexual activity between teenagers or other unmarried people. No way. No how.

Sometimes we could head off our children's challenges of our value system, sometimes we had to trust their divergences as right for them. Just as my own belief system reflects that of my parents, it is not without modifications and adjustments. I expect nothing different from my children, although I hope they will retain the best of the value system carved in the heart of our home.

And they will always have each other to confer with on these decisions. One of the blessings of raising children is watching their relationships with one another evolve from sometimes rivalrous siblings to playmates to close friends. It is not unlike the relationship I had with my own brother. Carl is almost four years younger than I am. When we were very young, we had only each other as playmates and I'm afraid Carl, being younger, got the worst end of that deal. I'd like to say that my kind and loving nature forbore any sibling rivalry between us and that he never had to suffer an older sister's harassment, but it simply wouldn't be true. I can remember sharing a room with him when we were very little. I had the top bunk and he had the bottom. I'd whisper at night, long after we were supposed to be asleep, "Carl, do you want to join my club?" "Sure," he'd answer. "Well," I'd continue, "you have to do. . . ." and I'd rattle off a list of absurd behaviors like running around the room four times, singing two lines of a song, and hopping back into bed without getting caught. He'd set off on his mission and in one out of three cases he'd get caught. I hid my head under my pillow, quietly laughing, as my dad marched into our room to reprimand my poor brother.

Long before the arrival of television, Carl and I played cowboys while riding Mom's brooms around the yard. We had our own version of Hide and Seek and Mother May I. We daydreamed for hours as we browsed through the Sears catalog and wrote make-believe shopping lists. In the fall we jumped into piles of leaves. In the winter, after stomping trails through the snow, we chugged our way over them, imagining ourselves to be little trains traveling on tracks.

Our house had a small vestibule leading into the living room. Carl and I often pretended we were two mechanics heading off to work and that vestibule was our elevator. With the handles of our toothbrushes in our mouths in mock imitation of pipe smokers, we called ourselves Mike and Mike and rode our "elevator" to the ground floor where the day's work awaited us. Lying under the seats of the kitchen chairs, we fancied ourselves repairing vehicles. Many years later as Dennis and I left our wedding reception, Carl handed me two small toothbrushes and toasted, "May all your problems be little ones and may they have as much fun playing Mike and Mike as we did!"

Like Carl and me, my kids relied on each other as playmates, confidantes, and companions. Rebecca and Rachel both looked up to and imitated their older brother. When Rebecca was in fourth grade, she wrote the following:

The Person I Admire the Most

> The person I most admire is not rich or on television; he is my big (big) brother. Jason is who I have always wanted to be like because he is so "good." Jason is one of the nicest people. He never fights with me, but he sometimes play fights. He always helps and never disobeys my parents. He doesn't swear either. Jason will give me help whenever I want it. He will play catch with me or even play basketball with me. If I am hurt or just feeling down, he will come up to my room, knock on the door, and ask if I am all right. Many people say bad things about their older brothers and sisters, but the only way I could say something like that about Jason was if I made it up. I really love my older brother.

When Jason left for his first year at Dartmouth, both girls missed him terribly. When he returned home for the first time, they cleaned his room, changed his sheets, and waited impatiently for his arrival. Jason, in turn, affirmed his role of older brother with good-natured humor and teasing.

It was common for Den and me to hear the girls chattering together in their room at night about their day's happenings. They helped each other study, and I was grateful that they had each other whenever they were disciplined. Behind the closed door of their room, they had free license to vent and to rage about their unjust parents. Today they call and visit each other frequently, offer moral support, and are quick to say "I love you."

I suspect that they still complain about Mom and Dad on occasion as well.

★ 5 ★

The Home Team

★ *REBECCA*

As the buzzer sounded, I took off running. I ran past Kara, Pam, Jamelle, Jennifer, and Carla. When I got to the end of the court, I turned around and saw most of my team in the center of the court hugging each other. Jamelle was alone at the free throw line. I ran to her and put my arms around her. Then I ran into the center and lost myself in giving hugs to everyone and jumping for the sheer joy of it. Coach Auriemma was leaping up and down before going over to shake the hand of Pat Summit, the coach of the other team. He joined us at center court and gave everybody hugs. We took turns cutting the net down and, despite his half-hearted cries of "Put me down!", we put him on our shoulders and carried him off the floor. He was ecstatic, glowing, happy, like everyone else on the team. We answered questions from the press, we took a congratulatory call from President Clinton, and we went back to the locker room. We didn't even have time to shower for the trophy ceremony. When we sat down for dinner at the hotel three hours later, we still wore our warm-ups and sweaty ponytails.

After we won the championship, we were asked constantly what it felt like to be down by six points at halftime. Reporters wanted to know what was going through our heads during the game. They wanted to know what it felt like when the buzzer sounded signifying the end of the game. They wanted to pass on to their readers the feeling of excitement and exhilaration we felt. I guess many people wanted to get as close as they could to the championship feeling. Can words really express how we felt? We were obviously excited and happy and every other good emotion there is.

Perhaps the best way for me to communicate my feelings is by showing a picture of my expression as I sprinted around. The amazing thing is that Jamelle had a very different look on her face, as did Jen and Pam and Kara and Coach Auriemma. Someone who didn't play or the teammate who was sitting on the bench when the buzzer sounded will feel differently. But we all had a common emotion. It's achieved when a group of people strive as hard as they possibly can toward a goal, sacrificing their bodies and their hearts, to achieve a dream.

To convey what winning meant to me, I'd have to go back and describe the hours I spent shooting hoops in my family driveway. I'd have to recall the years of practice, bus trips, airplane departure lounges, and baggage pick-ups. I'd remember the moment during the Virginia game my junior year when I first heard a crowd go wild while I was playing. (Was this when I began to emerge as a real basketball player?) During that game, for the first time we put ourselves to the test: "Our team is pretty good and Virginia has a great reputation. So how good are we? Let's see."

And, once I'd recounted all that and reached my final season with the UConn Huskies, I'd have to describe the game against Tennessee. It was a home game. That night Gampel Pavilion was sold out. We'd had sellouts before, but this time people were packed to the rafters. Some people were even scalping tickets. The fans were electric.

We were staying in a hotel because we were on winter break and the dorms were closed. The night before the game, one team member said, "We could be the number one ranked team in the country if we beat Tennessee." This seemed like an amazing realization, and the proverbial light went on in our heads. Kara Wolters came in, jumped on my bed and told me how nervous she was. But anyone who knows Kara knows that, as Coach Auriemma puts it, she makes coffee nervous.

I missed the first shot I took in that game. After I missed it, I told myself that the game I was playing now wasn't any different from any other game. Before that moment, I had been a bit apprehensive because it was Tennessee, and in women's basketball, Tennessee is *the* name. Five minutes later, Jen Rizzotti grabbed us all by our shirts, pulled us into a huddle, and screamed at us to get our act together because we *were* going to win this game. I knew then that we were going to win. From that point on I was flying. Nearly everyone on the team did something we really needed. As Tennessee repeatedly made runs at us down the stretch, Kara scored a crucial basket or Nykesha Sales made a great steal. Whether there were important shots to be made, rebounds to be grabbed, or in-your-face defense to be played, everyone stepped up to the challenge.

The crowd backing us made more noise than any crowd I'd ever heard. They simply did not let us lose the game. They stood in their seats, screamed, clapped, hollered, and did anything else they could to make noise. They helped make this game one of the best experiences I ever had playing basketball. Just looking around after the final buzzer sounded and seeing people jumping up and down and hugging each other because their team had won defined for me what sports is all about. It's a tremendous feeling that goes way beyond the feelings shared by the team. It's felt by anyone cheering for the home team. In some cases, it's felt by anyone watching the game. It was definitely there during this game on January 16. Well, the feeling that I had running down the court in Minneapolis after the final buzzer of the championship game felt something like that.

The feeling of victory after the Final Four lasted until the end of the next day. After speaking with the press, we met our families in the hallway outside our locker room. As we navigated the gauntlet of hugs, word was passed around that there was to be a postgame meal and party back at the hotel. After grabbing as much Final Four paraphernalia as is legally allowed, we loaded the bus. After my shower, I called some friends back in Connecticut and learned that the media was broadcasting a celebratory pickup game taking place in our family driveway in Southwick. My father called the police to tell them to keep an eye on the house only to find out that the police had told the media where we lived. We cheered the news broadcasts announcing our victory and then put our parents to bed. We were staying at a hotel on the outskirts of Minneapolis and I think the idea was that no press would be around. With that in mind, we partied long and hard throughout the night.

When we arrived back in Connecticut, we began to feel a million new emotions. There were thousands of people waiting for us at the airport, thousands of people lining the roads home, thousands of people on campus. When you win a championship, at first you simply enjoy the feeling that surrounds you. The following day, you begin to celebrate what you've done. Then suddenly, the feeling separates from you. It becomes something that happened, something in the past. After a while, I just longed to be away from all the commotion. I wanted to have a chance to think, to put all the emotions away for a while, and just rest.

My teammates remember different things about that season. We laugh about the look on Kara's face the day Coach kicked her out of practice. We recall sitting behind the North Carolina State cheerleaders and watching their men play as we laughed at Jamelle standing on her chair trying to do the cheers herself. We joke about the many faces of Missy Rose during our morning workouts. We remember what it felt like to sit in

Coach's room at 2:30 A.M. in Minneapolis and watch a tape of our national championship victory won only twelve hours before while Jen slept in a chair with a banner tied around her head. To the players, the season was much more than the games we won or the long hours of practice. It was about the friendships and love we had for each other. It was about twelve individuals learning how to be a family.

We weren't always the team that we were my senior year. My relationship with Coach Auriemma changed dramatically over the four years I was in college. When I was a freshman, I looked up to him in a lot of ways, but I didn't always understand him. I didn't understand why he yelled at me in practice or why he made the decisions he did. Then again, I was only eighteen years old. My sophomore year was probably the hardest year for me in terms of basketball. Because of injuries and a player who had quit, there were only eight people on the team. We were a decent team, we just didn't have the numbers. This meant there was more pressure on me to do well. I'd play okay in one game and poorly the next, and I couldn't blame my inconsistencies on being a freshman. Generally, this sort of responsibility and pressure doesn't come until you're a junior or senior. It knocked on my door when I was a sophomore.

My relationship with Coach during my sophomore year became pretty strained, too. When you're unhappy about the way you are playing, you become sensitive. This sensitivity combined with being yelled at all the time by your coach is a losing combination, however you look at it. It seemed to me that Coach was yelling at me every day in practice and pointing out every little miscue. I thought that he was constantly questioning my effort. I began to dread going to practice because I knew when it was over I was going to feel terrible. And I held Coach responsible for that. Feeling mistreated and misunderstood, I didn't try to understand his point of view or temper my reactions to what he said. After Christmas, it got so bad that we walked past each other in the hall after practice and, without uttering a word, we both looked the other way.

The evening after I passed Coach in the hall, our associate head coach, Chris Dailey, "kidnapped" Pam Webber and me and took us to Coach's house. The idea was to sit down and discuss the problems we were having. I basically let Coach do all the talking and didn't say a word. He told me that he had been coaching a certain way for many years and that he was not going to change. I had to learn how to play for him. I found it difficult to come out and say what I was thinking. On the way home in the car, I complained, "He's always questioning my effort; the problem isn't my effort all the time." I went on and on until we got back to the hotel. When we pulled up, Coach Dailey said, "Well, why didn't you tell him all that?" I wasn't sure. But before I went to bed, I gathered my thoughts and called him up. I told him I wanted to meet with him in his office the next day.

During our meeting I told him that I hated the way he constantly questioned my commitment. He listened and then told me exactly what he wanted from me as a player. He said that the reason he got so frustrated was that he watched me do something really well one moment and then completely wrong the next. He took me to task, he said, because he knew what I was capable of and he was impatient to see me reach my potential. If you play great one day and poorly the next, the problem can't be anything but concentration; it's your head rather than your skills. As soon as I understood that he was simply trying to get the most out of me, my anger at him disappeared. My mind cleared. A defining change in our relationship occurred that day. We still joke about the night CD "kidnapped" Pam and me and held us hostage at Coach's house. I guess you could say we've come a long way since that cold day in January!

Coach Dailey provided an altogether different challenge. One of the things we had to put up with while playing at Connecticut was Coach Dailey's set of regulations. Most of these had absolutely nothing to do with basketball. They involved the proper ways to behave, dress, and conduct ourselves, especially on road trips. She was, in every sense, the fashion police! Her biggest pet peeve was the team walking around with Walkmans on our heads. She thought this was tacky and rude. As a result, we weren't allowed to wear headphones while walking anywhere in public. We could put them on only on the bus or plane and were allowed to wear them in airports only after arriving at our gate. If we were on the bus and she was making an announcement, we had to remove the headsets completely from our heads. It didn't matter if they were turned off. She wanted them away from our ears so she could be sure we were listening. Every freshman questioned this rule when she first arrived on campus, but CD never budged. I'm sure that if she is still coaching in twenty years, the Walkman rule will still be in place (assuming, of course, that Walkmans aren't a thing of the past).

She was also a big stickler about our dress code. We weren't allowed to wear jeans when traveling. We had to wear either skirts or dress pants, but the main rule was that we always had to be "neat." Even for home games we had to dress up. Jen and I often complained about this particular rule. After all, we arrived at games about two hours before they were to start and well before any fans were there. Usually we entered Gampel without a single eye upon us. After games, we spent time talking to the media and treating our injuries. By the time we emerged from the locker room in our "nice outfits," the only people there to greet us were our families. Everyone else had left long before. Jen and I laid this out before Coach Dailey but she just ignored us. Rules were rules and they were going to be obeyed. Even if it meant we had to walk back to our dorms at 11:00 P.M. in 30-degree weather over treacherous ice wearing slippery shoes and stockings (I am definitely exaggerating here).

* * * *

Femininity. Ever since I entered college I have heard questions about female athletes and femininity. The femininity of women athletes is always questioned, and, by extension, their sexuality. I'm glad I didn't really have to worry about this issue until I reached college, when I was old enough to not take those questions personally. Soon after I arrived, someone told me that she had a friend who was gay and was wondering about me. I was, like, *"What?"* And she said, "Well, she asked me if you were gay and if you were would you be interested in meeting her." It was all new to me; I couldn't figure out how I could have given someone the impression that I was gay. I even got a letter saying, "You display lesbian tendencies on the court. Are you gay?" And I thought, "Why does this person think I'm gay? Because I block shots or rebound a basketball?" It seemed incredible.

I don't want anyone to think I'm something I'm not. I don't want anyone to think I'm a lesbian in the same way I don't want anyone to think I'm a math whiz or someone who is hard to get along with. But it's not really the same thing. I know it shouldn't matter whether or not people think that I'm gay, but somehow it does. I hope I treat the gay people I know the same as I treat my other friends, but I guess there is a stigma attached to being gay that makes me shy away from the label even when I know it's not true. Is that being a hypocrite? Maybe. It's also something many female athletes are very sensitive about.

I guess people still consider team sports like basketball to be something masculine, although I don't know why. There's nothing masculine about being competitive. There's nothing masculine about trying to be the best at everything you do, nor is there anything wrong with it. I don't know why a female athlete has to defend her femininity just because she chooses to play sports. Coach Dailey was aware of the stigma surrounding female athletes and wanted her team to put forth a different image. She knew that the only time most people saw us was when we were on the court wearing ponytails and sweating profusely. Most people didn't have a chance to see us the other twenty-two hours of the day, but for the few that did, Coach Daily wanted us to be prepared.

Some fans must have had the notion that we walked around all the time in our uniforms with our hair up and no makeup on, because they were always saying how much better my teammates and I looked off the court. We heard, "You look much prettier in person" all the time. I don't know if that meant we looked awful on the court or if it just shows that people sometimes can't see the woman behind the athlete. Maybe they are just reassured when they see a dress, or are relieved that we know how to do our hair and wear makeup. Not that Coach Dailey told us how to do our hair or to wear makeup. She simply told us we should put forth the image we wanted people to have of us.

I've never really enjoyed wearing makeup. Unlike Kara. Kara Wolters was known as Miss Mary Kay. Once I called her at home and her mom told me she was at a Mary Kay party, which is like a Tupperware party but with cosmetics instead of plastic containers. When she first visited UConn, she brought a gym bag filled entirely with cosmetics. Included was something called Stress Relief Spray, which Kara spent $8 on. It was a colorless, odorless liquid. To everyone else on the planet it was water. To Kara, a woman who frequently upholds the notion that Elvis is alive, it was Stress Relief Spray. It got worse after she arrived on campus. After working out, Kara took out her makeup bag—which was about the size of a suitcase—and started applying her beauty aids.

Kara is a big goof (I mean that with complete affection) who never ceases to amaze me. She's constantly improving her game, on court and off. As her confidence grew, she finally became proud of the fact that she is 6′7″. People stare at her, not because of her height, but because of her accomplishments. She deserves everything good that comes her way. She makes us laugh just by doing and saying bizarre things. She makes a mess in the locker room and is so messy that no one has been able to room with her for more than a year. But we all love her anyway.

I must admit that Kara does look really nice once she is done up. Still, I never had the time or patience to do to my face what she did to hers, despite all her efforts trying to convince me that hair spray and makeup were my friends. The one time I let my teammates do my makeup and hair was when I went to the ESPYs (ESPN's awards) near the end of my senior year. The ESPN award show was a black-tie affair and since I spent a lot of money on a nice gown, it was expected that my hair and make-up be a little more elaborate than normal. Unfortunately, I wasn't able to make an appointment at a hairdresser to get "done up." My teammates happily volunteered to be my fairy godmothers. Pam applied the makeup (Kara's, of course) and then proceeded to curl, spray, and pin my hair. It seemed like we had the whole team crammed into the dormitory bathroom witnessing the makeover. It took a good hour or more to complete the transformation. Pam didn't let me look in the mirror until she was finished. Naturally, when I finally saw myself, I was horrified; my hair was too high and my makeup too heavy. But after encouragement (and threats), I promised to leave it alone.

Everyone was excited for me and anxiously waited to see me in the gown. Coach Dailey and a few of my teammates brought cameras and took tons of pictures. Some girls who lived on my floor (even ones I didn't know very well) came out of their rooms and took pictures also. To this day, I haven't seen one of them. Anyway, once the limousine arrived, my teammates were like kids at a carnival. They all climbed in and out of the car and took even more pictures. I was just glad that the driver was patient and didn't mind these college women treating his automobile like a ride at the amusement park.

I must admit that I was tempted to remove some of the makeup on the ride to New York City, but I knew that if I got caught on camera without my "face" on (the award show was televised), my teammates would give me hell upon my return. So I didn't take any of the makeup off. I also didn't get on camera, which was a relief.

When I started making appearances on television shows and participating in photo shoots where there were professional makeup artists, I realized how makeup can enhance your looks without making you look like a painted doll. My mother had encouraged me throughout high school to go to someone and have my colors done so I would know which color clothes are most flattering, which color makeup to wear, and how to put it on. I've been so busy that I've yet to do this, but I do want to look the best I can off the court. I admit that perhaps some occasions call for a little more makeup than I'm accustomed to. I still don't wear very much (especially in the summer when I have a tan), but I'm also no longer so completely opposed to having it on. One nice thing is that my boyfriend says he likes it when I don't wear much makeup because he thinks I am beautiful naturally. (No matter how high your self-esteem is, that's always nice to hear.)

Maybe sometime soon I will finally get my coloring done and make my mother happy. But I doubt it will ever be as normal a routine as, for example, working out. Thank God I have learned the benefits of a more natural and tamer hairstyle on my own. That's saved me a lot of time. Looking back at my high school pictures I wish I had had more direction in those matters. My mother had encouraged me to get a hairstyle that was a little more refined than the wild locks curled and sprayed on my head, but like any other self-respecting teenager, I thought I had better ideas about fashion than my mother. I'm sorry to say I did not.

One thing I've never questioned is my femininity. No matter how my makeup and hair looked, I always felt very comfortable with myself, even in "boys' clothes." When I'm not playing basketball, I like to wear earrings. I rarely wear perfume. I don't wear my hair in a high ponytail when I'm off the court; usually it's down or pulled back at the base of my neck. I only braid it for games. I feel most glamorous when I dress up for black-tie affairs. I wear heels(!) and stockings, my hair is done, and I have makeup on, but I'm just as happy after practice when I'm walking around in warm-ups. Too often, particularly when we're young, other people's ideas about what femininity is can become our own.

Whatever femininity is, it doesn't have anything to do with how much you weigh or how popular you are with boys. It would, of course, be best if we didn't have to confront such questions at all, if we could be as oblivious to them as the men's basketball team seems to be. I would tell my hypothetical little sister, "If people on the outside question you, don't let it bother you. Just put their questions out of your head." Hopefully, people will start to realize that you can be an athlete and a woman. Women are out there proving that every day. I think our UConn team proved that, and I think the National Team is proving that too. We're promoting the idea that womanhood and athletics are complementary. Fortunately, I never thought that combination was a bad thing. Thank God.

And, although it was a hassle at times, I am glad Coach Dailey enforced her rules about dress. Whenever our team went to banquets, we always looked nice. (My fifth grade teacher would probably have been shocked at my transformation!) By making sure we were well turned out, Coach Dailey was trying to undermine the expectations people seemed to have about female athletes. Although it might have been easier at times to just throw on a sweat suit for the flight to an away game, CD gave us a different image to think about. In the end, it's up to us to defeat these attitudes. By dressing up, we increased our power of persuasion and strengthened our sense of self. Looking back, I think we all thank Coach Dailey for that.

It's kind of funny. Even though CD is no longer there to monitor my wardrobe or my wearing a Walkman, her ideas have become my own. I will never walk around in public with a headset on and I am conscious of how I'm dressed when I'm traveling. I don't wear jeans to games. Once you establish a habit, it becomes hard to break, regardless of whether it has anything to do with femininity or reversing stereotypes. I think I learned some pretty good habits from my coaches at UConn.

* * * *

Like any freshman, I was nervous when I first entered college. I didn't know what to expect from basketball, from classes, or anything else. It was my first time away from home. But I was better off than most because I had teammates who looked out for me and who took care of me. The coaches decided to have me room with Pam Webber.

When we first met, I didn't think we had very much in common. In reality, however, we were both laid back and had similar ideas about what was important in life. We hit it off very well from the beginning, although we were both freshman and, by definition, didn't know much about college life. The person who taught me was a senior on our team, Meghan Pattyson. If she went out on the weekend, she made sure to include us. Whenever there was a party, she asked if we wanted to go. It must have been hard for her to constantly include us, especially since we were underage and most places wouldn't admit us. She did, anyway, and most of the people I met that year were her friends; I wonder if I would have met anyone without her.

That was freshman year. As it turned out, Pam and I roomed together for the next three as well. We never really got into a big fight or argument. We talked nonstop and shared almost everything that was going on in our lives. Sometimes we just lay in our lofts and talked for hours before we went to sleep. Sometimes we watched TV or listened to music. Our relationship worked out pretty well that way: She owned the CD player and I owned all the CDs, she owned the couch and I owned the fridge. Her mom even bought us matching comforters for our beds. We used those same comforters all the way through to graduation.

Come exam time, I stressed out and studied as much as I could. I was the sort who read every book on the syllabus and attended every class. I was known among the other athletes at school for being a nerd. "Where were you last night, Lobo? At the *library?*" It amazed me sometimes how few people attended classes until exam time came around. I could always be counted on to have the notes from every lecture, but I never trusted anyone's notes but my own. So there I was, cramming for exams in our dorm room while Pam was napping. Yet when grades came out, hers were nearly always better. I could never figure out how she managed that.

When I was home, even just for one day, I talked to Pam on the phone. It drove Mom crazy. The conversations lasted at least an hour. My mother couldn't understand why I needed to talk to someone for so long if I was going to see her the next day. But that was just the way it was. Besides, anyone who knows Pam realizes that, for her, there is no such thing as a short phone conversation. During our marathon late-night conversations we talked about everything; we even made plans to live in the same cul-du-sac when we got married (whether or not that happens remains to be seen). I do know one thing, however; my phone bill will have plenty of charges to her for the rest of my life. Everything I learned from and about Pam in our four years together was a good thing.

My other close friend on the team was Jen Rizzotti. She was a year behind me, so we only had three years to spend together. Since Pam liked to stay in with her boyfriend on the weekends, and I enjoyed going out, I could always count on Jen to go with me. Just about every weekend Jen and I and a bunch of our teammates would jump into a car to go dancing or something. If people saw me out, they knew Jen was somewhere nearby and vice versa. If she needed anything from me, I had no problem rearranging other plans in order to help her. I didn't think twice about it because I always knew she would do the same for me.

Jen was the person I told most of my problems to. She's a great listener and tells you how she feels no matter what. We spent many hours in her room just hanging out and talking. She is one of the most loyal friends I have ever had. You can count on her in any situation. She is exactly the same way on the court, extremely reliable. On road trips we would room together, because Jen asked the assistant coach to put us together when she was making the rooming list. Before or after a game, I knew who she wanted to talk to on the phone and who she didn't; if it were someone important to her and I was on the phone already, I would gladly get off. We understood and respected each other. I always knew that if she gave her word on something, it would get done.

She looked out for me constantly. If I got hurt by someone's actions, she was hurt. If I was upset or mad at someone, Jen had a hard time not feeling the same way. I was her friend and she cared what other people did or said to me. She treated all her close friends exactly the same. She doesn't know how to be any different. A friend like her only comes around once in a lifetime.

Missy Rose is a teammate who deserves a lot of credit. She worked incredibly hard at practice but was not always rewarded with playing time during games. She is a fun kid to be around and someone I truly miss. She is quick to show affection, and doesn't bite her tongue if she finds something unjust. She handles our jokes about her tight jeans with good-natured demeanor (usually) and doesn't try to hide the fact that she *hates* early morning. Coach affectionately called her Sibyl because she had so many different personalities, depending on the time of day. During the two years I played with her, she earned my complete respect. She works so hard both on and off the court. She's a great friend, and that never changes, no matter what the time of day.

Then there is Jamelle Elliott. I *love* Jamelle. Off the court she's like a teddy bear, and on the court she is the most aggressive player imaginable. She's physical, and if you're not on her team, she'll just beat you up and do whatever she can to win. Then, when you step off the court, she's your best friend. She'll hug you and make you smile before you realize what's happened. It totally baffled me how she could just switch it on and off. Most of the time the crowd or fans see you as the person you are on the court. If they never met Jamelle off the court, they'd never know who she really is.

I think if you talked to any basketball player, she would say she was two different people on and off the court. To be a good player, you have to be aggressive and ready to physically punish your opponent. When you step off the court, you have to have the ability to be friends with those same people. To be the best player I can be, I need to be, as Coach Auriemma always said, an SOB on the court. When I see someone take a cheap shot at one of my teammates, my first reaction—if no one is looking—is to run down the court and exact justice. If she were going up for a rebound, I might legally elbow her in a way that wouldn't be called a foul or look cheap. That's not a dirty play, and I don't do things like that often, but I have to "send the message" that I won't let her get away with doing anything to my teammates. I've never actually hurt anyone, but I have given them something to think about. Coach always told me I was too nice on court, that I shouldn't hang back and wait for a cheap shot at a teammate to get fired up because that won't happen in every game. To take my game to another level, I have to want to dominate people, both physically and emotionally, as soon as I step on the court. I have to be more like Jamelle.

I love this "in-control" feeling, and, when it finally kicks in, I'm entirely possessed. The opportunity to appease this side of my nature is pure joy. If you're like me and want to be a good person, sports lets you be aggressive on the court and get away with it. Other women might save it for the corporate boardroom! But, as yet, it's just not something I can switch on, no problem; something still has to happen to fire me up! To be the best, I need to be able to make it happen on my own, like Jamelle. As a healthy outlet for aggression and competitiveness, I recommend sports for everyone, even if you're just a fan. You release as much aggression in the stands. Just watch my mother!

After the Tennessee game, attention paid to the Connecticut women's basketball program increased incredibly. Everyone seemed to be interested in doing a story on the UConn Huskies. Each and every time, the stories talked about us as athletes, women, and positive role models. We made the network news, ESPN, the *New York Times,* and many other national media outlets. At the end of the season, we had far more media requests than Barb Kowal in athletic communications could fill. We had to start saying no to some people and giving time limits to others. Practices became closed to the media for the first time. Things were changing but the changes were necessary. We were now ranked number one in the country and had captured the hearts of many basketball fans in the state of Connecticut. Jen and I joked after the Tennessee game that if we got pulled over that evening for speeding while driving to the Harford Civic Center for the men's game, there was no way a cop would give us a ticket. Luckily, we didn't have to find out if our theory was true.

The night after the Tennessee game and after our men's game against Georgetown, we went back to the hotel. Anyone who called our room heard cheerful voices answer, "We're number one, how may we help you?" We were definitely on cloud nine. We had to come back down to earth quickly, however, since we had practice the next day for a game two days later against Boston College.

The media in Connecticut has been described as "the horde" because it is so large. During my senior year we had four local television stations and countless newspapers covering our every move on the court. Fortunately, just about all the press we got was positive. I didn't mind giving interviews because all of the reporters were so upbeat. I guess it's hard to be negative when a team doesn't lose. I think, too, that the journalists covering us didn't think people would tire of reading positive articles. But I swear there are skeptics everywhere. In most sports coverage there is usually someone out there trying to stir up negative press; sometimes they find something and sometimes they don't.

For example, at one point during my senior year, both the men's and women's teams at UConn were ranked number one in the country. Inevitably, one of the questions reporters asked once the men dropped from their spot was, "Do the men resent your success?" or, "What is the relationship like between the men's and women's teams?" I almost think they were hoping for controversy. They didn't realize how supportive the two teams are of each other. We would have liked nothing better than to have the men be national champions, and they treated us with the same respect. They came to our games and cheered us on; we went to theirs. This wasn't always easy, however, because the men were always swamped by autograph seekers and couldn't watch the game without interruptions. Later in the season, we got the same treatment at their games. It got to the point where we spent more time signing autographs than looking at the players on the court. Like everyone else in Connecticut, we didn't feel that their success would take away from ours.

The coverage of the Boston College game, too, went a little sour. I personally played awfully and our team got off to a really slow start. Afterwards, Coach Auriemma was caught on camera criticizing the officials and the way the other team played. Of course, all of this was covered on the nightly news and in the newspapers the next day.

What didn't show up on the nightly news from Coach Auriemma's press conference, however, was what really mattered. After the game I was walking behind Coach to the media room. The press had been told repeatedly that we would answer questions once we got to the press conference, no sooner. I was miserable. Reporters were shouting questions at me as I walked by them. When we got into the media room, I had to answer questions about why I played so poorly and what had happened to me. Before letting me answer, Coach interrupted by remarking on the poor officiating and the fact that the other team was trying to beat me up instead of simply stopping me. I don't know what kind of impression these comments made on people reading their morning paper or watching the evening news. I know, however, they were coming from a man who was trying to protect his players.

Now, when I talk about Coach Auriemma, I say that other than my family, he has probably had the biggest influence on me. He has taught me the importance of getting the most out of myself and, more important, how to do so. I learned what it really means to work hard and that my definition of hard work is constantly changing. The basketball player I am today is a direct result of his and our other coaches' work. Coach also showed me how to handle different situations in life. Just watching how he deals with the media and listening to him speak in front of groups is entertaining. He has a great sense of humor and uses it constantly. He treats people with respect and commands it for himself. I simply have a lot to thank him for. I've done so many times publicly but it will never be enough. Basically, I just enjoy being around him. That is, when he's not yelling at me to pass the ball or calling me the "worst post player in America." I guess everyone has his moments.

Role models can be slippery things. While I was growing up, the only role models I looked to were my parents and my brother and sister. It was that straightforward: I decided what was right and wrong by watching my parents. They didn't teach through words alone but constantly reinforced what they said through their actions. They talked about the value of hard work and then came home every night and did their work after dinner. They talked about the value of love and then showered it upon their children every chance they got. They showed each of their children how to live honestly. As a result, there was no need for me to look elsewhere for role models.

I recognize now that a lot of people don't have the advantage of a stable home like I had and often look to sports stars for direction. That is when a role model can become slippery. Of course, I too had favorite baseball, football, and basketball players when I was growing up. I liked the way Larry Bird played, and I remember hearing a story or two about how he was such a hard worker, but I didn't *really* know him. And even though I may have wanted to model my game after his, I always wanted to model who I was as a person after my parents. Both of my parents were always there. I only "knew" the athletes when they were on the court or field, whereas I knew my parents in every aspect of their lives. They never fought and rarely argued, at least not in front of us kids. It was a blessing that my parents were both teachers, because it allowed them to have the same schedule as their children. We always ate dinner together and took family vacations every summer. The jobs they had really allowed us to be a close family. Since sports was only a part of my life, I needed good examples of how to live right, and my parents provided those examples.

When I got to UConn I found other role models. I learned different lessons from every person on that team, as well as from Coach Dailey and Coach Auriemma. I would consider both of them my role models. A team like ours does not come along very often. Not just because we went 35-0, but because there was something special about the way we were a true TEAM. Of course we had problems like any other team. We had squabbles among team members and small arguments off the court (never fighting over Kara's Stress Relief Spray, of course!). However, just like a family, we ate together, went out together, and spent time together, not because we were told to but because we wanted to. Don't get me wrong; everyone did her own thing and spent time with her boyfriends and other friends from class. But when all was said and done, we were a family. We stuck up for each other through thick and thin. Someone on the team could pick on Kara or make fun of the way she was wearing her hair that day, but if we heard anyone else doing it, we would get ticked off, just like on the basketball court. If a player on the opposing team gave Pam a cheap shot or anything that resembled one, she had better look out because Jamelle was going to kill her the next time down the floor with a *legal* screen. If someone elbowed Kara or me, she had to beware because sooner or later Jen would be sure to strip the ball out of her hands or dribble by her, making her look like a fool. Everyone looked out for each other, especially on the court. It was how we played. It was the only way we knew how to play.

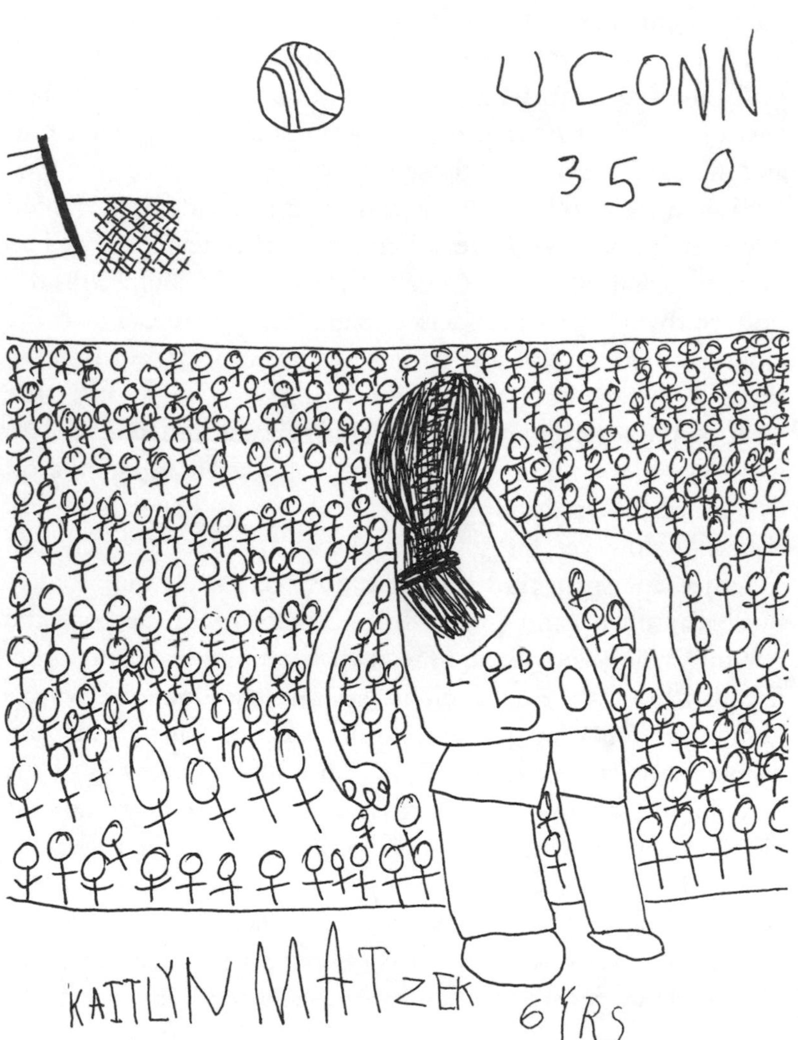

★ 6 ★

Tall in Love

★ *RUTHANN*

My fantasies of romance were born with the rise of rock 'n' roll. The lyrics on 45-rpm records wooed my adolescent imagination. Long before I was old enough to date, my baby-sitting money purchased the latest and greatest of the top twenty. My very first investment was "A Rose and a Baby Ruth" by George Hamilton IV. Unlike today's songs that are permeated with raw sex, "Love Me Tender" and "Where The Boys Are" titillated our wildest dreams with the promise of a kiss and love everlasting. Sitting on my bed listening to the slow ballads of the day for mood music, I immersed myself in the trials and tribulations of the heroines in *Wuthering Heights, Little Women,* and *Gone with the Wind.*

Without the access to the cars, phones, malls, and cinemas that kids have today, my friends and I gathered at each other's houses and gossiped endlessly about the boys of our dreams. My first crush was on a boy over whom I was truly head and shoulders taller. Dubbed by the kids as Beanpole, Stringbean, and Turnpike ("you can go for miles without a curve in sight"), I paid little attention to the fact that I was taller than just about everyone in my class. Social life outside of school centered around parties where dancing and occasional kissing games like Spin the Bottle took place.

Couples were the exception in our school, but I envied those girls with boyfriends, wishing I were prettier, funnier, or whatever in order to capture the attention of the object of my affection at the moment. One boy won my heart in junior high, and he remained the focus of my desires throughout high school. I am embarrassed to admit that I pursued him unabashedly and suspect I frightened him right out of his mind! I did childish things that now, of course, I know don't work: I sent notes, I sent friends, I sent looks and smiles and—I sent him scurrying!

After four years of daydreaming about this young man, I was informed via the grapevine that he was planning to invite me to our senior prom. I couldn't believe it! After I heard, the first thing I had to do, I'm ashamed to say, was disinvite the boy I was seeing from another town. To do this, I concocted a story about how the shyest, most retiring kid in my class had asked me to go. "If I turn him down," I said, "I will scar him for life." Then I impatiently hung around the phone waiting for THE CALL. At last it came. Standing in the kitchen wearing my slip, I gushed out my acceptance, and after replacing the receiver, I danced around the room in disbelief and excitement. As my parents drove into the driveway, I waltzed out the door, still in my slip, and announced to the world that fairy tales do come true.

Although I had a lovely senior prom evening, I learned a lesson I have carried with me ever since. My date was truly a nice person, but it was a struggle to carry on a conversation. The young man to whom I had devoted hours of thought and earnest affection didn't exist, and the romantic fantasy I had nurtured over the years collapsed. Every time a student confides an unrequited love in my counseling office, I am reminded of my first "love."

Traipsing off to a small Connecticut college, one hundred miles from home, I looked forward to meeting new people, and like most college students, to living away from home for the first time. At the same time I reluctantly left behind a summer romance. The night before my departure, after our good-byes and goodnight kiss, I entered the house crying. "I know what it feels like," my mother said, abandoning her usual homilies about being strong. "If it's meant to be, then things will work out." She comforted me with a hug.

My first year in college was uneventful. I lived off campus with my roommate in the home of a professor and his family. Although I had been a National Honor Society student in high school, I was terrified that I wouldn't make the grade in college. Most of my first year I spent studying diligently and writing letters to my boyfriend. I listened to Shelley Fabares sing "Johnny Angel" countless times and longed to be back home.

I moved into a dormitory for sophomore year. I did not know that my life was about to change significantly. On a Friday night in late September, I accompanied my roommates to a dance held in the women's gym. As was my custom, I scanned the crowd to see if there were any men whose heads were at least at the same height as mine or higher. I spotted a tall, lean fellow with jet black hair styled in a crewcut. He bore a serious, contemplative look on his face. The collar of his khaki jacket was turned upward, a la James Dean. I wrote him off, thinking, "He looks like a hood!"

The following evening our dormitory was sponsoring a block hop. As a member of the dance committee, I volunteered to man the refreshment table. My attention was attracted to a young man named Cliff who stopped by the table for coffee. To my dismay, he was interested in my roommate, Sue, and I in turn was introduced to none other than "the hood" I had spotted the night before! With little enthusiasm I accepted his invitation to dance.

"What did you say your name is?" I queried.

"Dennis Lobo," he responded.

"Ovo?" I repeated over the music.

"Lobo," he repeated.

"Obo?" I tried one more time.

"Lobo," he stated in frustration. Not wanting to appear the complete fool, I dropped it. I had noticed, however, that he had the most remarkable dark eyes, framed by the longest lashes.

Encouraged by his buddies, Dennis invited me to go for coffee with his friends and mine after the dance. When I arrived back at the dorm, I went to the phone book and looked up Obo and Ovo. "I knew it," I chided myself, "he was just giving me a line." That night, I complained to my roommates, "Look who you met tonight, and look who I ended up with!" Little did I know I was referring to the man who would become the anchor in my life.

Several days later, I spotted Dennis as I was leaving the building where I had just completed my phys. ed. class. He was busy chatting with some friends as he sauntered toward me. I quickly plunked myself down on the steps and adopted a casual air. As he approached, I looked up, caught his eye, and nonchalantly remarked, "So you do go here!"

Not too long after, a group of us decided to get together for coffee one evening. For college students in 1962 that meant six people driving two hours in a VW bug to a "nearby" college town. We got there around midnight; it seemed like we were nuts. To add insult to injury, on my return to campus, I couldn't get back into the dormitory. Knowing that I could be expelled for breaking the 9:30 curfew, I hurried back to the car and racked my brain for someplace to stay. I finally decided to return to the house I had lived in my freshman year, because I knew the doors were left unlocked and friends were renting my former room. Afraid of waking the entire household, I tiptoed upstairs and curled up on the floor where I slept until dawn. Before the rest of the house arose, I quietly exited and made a hasty retreat back to the dorm.

My mother would have killed me if she had known I was out after curfew. Just as she had when I was in high school, on my visits home she insisted on knowing my whereabouts. She considered "parking" much too dangerous, and filled my head with a variety of monstrous possibilities, including peeping Toms and serial killers preying on unsuspecting couples. Although she painted vivid pictures of wild beasts outside the car, her unspoken fears were really inspired by the dangers within. "If you want to go parking, come home and park in your own driveway." Of course when I tried that, about two minutes after we pulled into the driveway, my mother started flicking the outside light on and off until I went inside.

When Dennis came to visit, she made certain we were chaperoned. We sometimes stayed up late watching television, waiting for a private moment or two, but my mother always sat up with us. She often dozed, but some internal radar system alerted her the moment Dennis put his arm around my shoulder. One eye would open and Mom would make sure we were behaving before falling back to sleep. She guarded my virginity with the passion of a mother bear and would have purchased a chastity belt if she could have. She certainly would have slept more soundly.

Dennis and I dated throughout the next three years of college. Our youth, our inexperience, and the customs of the times combined for a sometimes rocky and tumultuous relationship. We quarreled over the silliest of things. If we were in a restaurant and I had the money, I wanted him to hand it to the waitress because in those days only men paid for dates. Dennis would refuse. Once, in the middle of a tiff, he and my roommate's boyfriend drove to a sorority dance in her car. Beside ourselves with jealousy and rage, Carole and I drove to the hall where the dance was taking place and crept around the building to peek in the windows. There were the guys having a good time! In retaliation, we found Carole's car in the parking lot and drove away, leaving the men to their own devices to get home.

Our quarrels were overshadowed, however, by the growing affection we felt for one another. Many a weekend morning I heard a plink on the window as Den stood outside the dorm tossing stones to wake me up. We studied together, drank coffee together, and munched on doughnuts in the car together. We sat for hours in the lounge sharing our dreams for the future, which gradually began to include each other. I am personally grateful that there were dormitory curfews; otherwise, I doubt I would have had the discipline to put studying before passion.

After three years of dating, we picked out the diamond. The jeweler unfolded a cloth containing loose diamonds that sparkled as they rested on the counter. One by one he set each stone apart as he described its individual merits. With excitement we made our selection, and the diamond was put on layaway. Every week Den made a payment on the diamond, and every week I quizzed him on how it looked in the setting I had not yet seen.

One evening in the spring of our senior year, Dennis invited me to go out to dinner. As we rode in the car to the restaurant, I asked him if he had seen the ring lately. "How does it look?" I badgered. "Why don't you see for yourself?" he replied as he tossed me a neatly wrapped box. Ripping open the package, I found my engagement ring. Den pulled under a street lamp in front of a fruit stand and ceremoniously asked me to marry him. I threw my arms around his neck and gave him a big kiss. As I opened my eyes I was horrified to see a group of young men standing by the fruit stand enjoying my open display of affection!

My mother's response to our engagement was less than enthusiastic. "That doesn't mean anything," she uttered over the phone when I called. I choked with anger. I wanted celebration and good wishes, but Mom gave me a wet blanket. But her insight into Den's and my relationship was keener than our own; four months after graduation, I returned the ring.

Den and I had both entered graduate school, but at two different universities, seventy miles apart. I was suddenly caught up in a social whirl I had never known before. For the first time in my life, offers to go out overwhelmed me. My head was turned and, by mutual consent, Dennis and I broke our engagement. Five months later, while getting ready for a date, I faced myself in the mirror and admitted that I didn't really want to go. The novelty of all the attention had waned. I hadn't met anyone for whom I truly cared. Getting into my car the following weekend, I made the two-hour trip to New Britain, Connecticut. I pulled into the driveway and Dennis came out of the house. I talked. He listened, reluctantly. I talked. He was skeptical. I talked. He said he'd give it a try. Two weeks later, the ring was back on my finger. This time my mother smiled. "I only wanted to know that you were sure," she said.

The first decade of our marriage laid the groundwork for a partnership that has sustained us ever since. We began our marriage with the values and expectations we had inherited from our families; sometimes those expectations were compatible and sometimes they were not. At first we did not have the wisdom or the experience to recognize and amicably resolve our differences. We grumbled, we pouted, we dug in our heels.

The task of adjusting to a new marriage was coupled with the task of adjusting to our teaching careers. Den had been hired to teach history in Granby, and I had been hired to teach elementary school at a state residential home. Our lives were further complicated by my first pregnancy. Within a year of our marriage, we were faced with lesson plans, homemaking, and morning sickness. My efforts to resolve these conflicts were made even more difficult by those feminists who had begun to chide women for choosing marriage and family over career. Having been raised by a woman who constantly conveyed the message that I could be whatever I wanted, I never questioned my decision to combine a career with marriage and family. Unlike some of my friends, I did not question that, after my God, it was my family and not my career that came first. I was angered by those women who suddenly appeared on television and the covers of magazines boldly pronouncing that those of us raising families were subservient, less fulfilled, and less important. I watched marriages of twenty and thirty years crumble as women, bombarded with the feminist message of the time and the general social upheaval, began to question the validity of their lives as mothers and homemakers. I had to contend with the challenges of a new marriage; I didn't need to be chastised by feminists as well.

To be fair, I have to laugh now at the suggestion by some politicians that women selfishly abandon their children to pursue the higher calling of their career. I was lucky, I liked teaching. It was not burning ambition that sent me back to the workforce six months after Jason was born, however. We simply could not have survived on one teacher's salary. When Rachel was born and Jason was nearly four, I decided to give domesticity my best shot and quit my job. To make ends meet, Den painted houses and worked tobacco during the summers. But before long, I was an Avon lady, hawking face creams from door to door. I know that the vast majority of working women are stuck in jobs where they are underpaid or overqualified. The problem for them is not how can they best fulfill their personal ambitions (though that is always nice), but how to keep bread on the table.

So I was caught in a net of confusion while trying to balance the demands of marriage and career. Dennis and I drew from two different frames of reference; his mother had been free to remain at home after the birth of her children, whereas my mother worked. The division of labor in each household was different. Often, serious differences between us found outlets through arguments over trifles. For example, during my growing up emptying the trash was a task relegated to the male members of my household; in Den's home, his mother did it. While each of us waited for the other to empty the trash, the trashcan bulged and overflowed. It became a test to see who would give in first. In my home, the person who used the bathtub was expected to scrub it. In Den's house, his mom did it. A major fight resulted when I discovered a dirty tub waiting for me. "Why should I clean up after you?" I bellowed. On the other hand, the thought of shoveling the snow or taking the car to the garage never crossed my mind; that was something my dad and brother did.

Den's mom, a headstrong and determined woman, balanced the raising of four children with the care and maintenance of a home, while my father-in-law, a practicing dentist, provided the income and managed the finances. My mom combined child rearing with her job as a cook in the local school system, and my dad, a builder and assessor, assumed some of the household chores like scrubbing the floor or doing the dishes. Thus, some of Den's and my expectations conflicted because our models were different. Our expectations clashed. Who should do the dishes? The shopping? Pay the bills? Is it your money? My money?

It would have been easy in those early years of our marriage to call it quits when faced with the aggravation of unresolved trashcan and bathtub grievances, as well as the reality of finances, child rearing, and housekeeping. I am grateful that social sanctions, strong family traditions, and our love for each other forced us to work through areas of disagreement. Seven years into our marriage, a colleague of ours returned from a church-sponsored Marriage Encounter. Normally witty, macho, and sarcastic, he described this weekend experience with gripping emotion and tear-filled eyes. I was moved by the change I sensed in him and discussed it with Den. We decided to attend a Marriage Encounter weekend as well. Secluded from the outside world, surrounded by couples committed to each other, we explored our relationship with each other and with God. We heard talks. We wrote letters to each other. We learned to communicate with greater understanding. I stopped assuming

Den could read my mind and he did the same. I became more willing to empty the trash and help with the shoveling. He became more willing to tackle dishes and pack the lunches. We shared our deepest thoughts and feelings. We left with a treasure of renewed commitment and faith. It was as if God moved from a Being "out there somewhere" to a Being housed in the core of my heart.

I heard on that Marriage Encounter weekend that the greatest gift a father can give to his children is to love their mother. My children have been blessed with such a father. Throughout our four-year courtship and almost thirty years of marriage, Den has been my partner in the unfolding of a deep and lasting love affair. An unselfish man, he has stood by my side through impetuous projects, fads of the moment, career challenges and changes. He has withstood my periodic attempts at playing the guitar and decorating. He held his tongue when an enormous antique jelly cupboard that he refused to purchase appeared in our living room unannounced. He supported my return to school for a second master's degree as well as my switch from classroom teacher to school counselor. He encouraged my run for the Southwick board of education and offered an occasional back rub when the challenges of that office overwhelmed me. He held me close in the stillness of the night as we faced together my diagnosis of a life-threatening disease.

Although these days his hairline is a little higher, the hair color remains jet black, a legacy from his mother. With a baseball cap casually pushed back from his brow, he can still melt my heart with those deep brown eyes and thick black lashes that captured my attention at that dance so many years ago. Only the varicose veins that tire his legs betray his youthful appearance and nature. I often catch a glimpse of the young man I fell in love with when a boyish grin of affection sweeps across his face. The smell of his skin and the touch of his cheek rekindle the passion and excitement of newly discovered love.

I have often wished for my children the love I have found with their father. He has made me feel special each day of our life together. He tells me he loves me in a myriad of ways: through words, notes, kisses, and hugs. In the heat of the summer, he makes me iced tea; in the cold of the winter, he kindles a fire in the wood-burning stove to warm the kitchen before I arise. In all the years we have been married, he has never once voiced disapproval of my hair style, my fashion, my makeup, or my figure. He drops in to see me in my office during the day and teases me with affection. In my worst moments he embraces me with love and compassion. He asks nothing in return. He is my rock, my foundation, my soul mate, the love of my life.

★ *REBECCA*

On my twenty-first birthday my parents and sister came up to school and took me out to dinner to celebrate. During the course of the meal, my parents told the stories of how they met, little fights they had, and other tidbits about their relationship before they got married. Some of the stories we'd heard before, others were completely new. Either way, my parents told them as if reliving them. The gleam and look in my mother's eye as she glanced at my father painted more of a picture than words ever could. The look my father gave back expressed more love than saying "I love you" a thousand times over.

When we were kids my sister and I used to say "oooh yuck" whenever my parents used to kiss in front of us. The summer after my mother was diagnosed with cancer, I went with the UConn team to Europe and my parents followed. I only got to see them for one day, but I took this wonderful picture of them walking down the crooked streets of Venice, holding hands. In the past they had never been so openly romantic. But after the cancer they both realized that life is short and you have to make the most of every day. My sister once happened to call mom about a half hour after my father returned from a six-week visit to Japan. She was rattling along about something or other when my mom said she had to get off the phone. Rachel had a few more things to say. My mother became more insistent. "Rachel, Dad and I are both standing here naked!" Rachel laughed and prattled on and might have continued indefinitely if she hadn't been interrupted by a dial tone.

During my birthday celebration I understood that although the woman who sat next to me was my mom and would always be, she was equally her mother's daughter, her husband's wife, and a young woman just like me. I don't know why it took me so long to see her this way. "I hope that you find someone who loves you as much as your father loves me," she told us that evening.

When she spoke these words I was beginning my senior year in college. However, even though I was twenty-one, I'd never been in love. I'd had boyfriends and dates, but I'd never truly fallen for someone. I couldn't begin to think about marriage or having a family. I didn't exactly worry about this, but every once in a while, I'd ask myself, "When am I ever going to meet the someone?"

I don't think I had higher expectations than other girls. I could hardly even say what I thought "love" actually was. I did know that when people, after a couple of weeks or a month of being with someone, said "Oh, I'm in love," it wasn't true. It takes longer than that to know. I may not have known what being in love was all about, but I knew it was more than going on a few dates. What I knew of "love," I learned from my parents' marriage. I saw how they treated each other. I expected and still expect to be treated at least as well as my father treats my mother. I know, too, that I'll love and respect my "true love" equally in return.

I had a few boyfriends growing up. My first kiss came in the sixth grade when I was "asked out" by the shortest boy in our class. We made an interesting couple because I was the tallest girl in the whole junior high. We were at a roller-skating rink sitting on the benches and he really wanted to kiss me. He pressed, "Let's kiss, let's kiss." I didn't really want to, but I gave in. After we kissed, I said to myself, "I don't want to do that again, that wasn't any big deal." To him I said, "Let's go back out and *skate.*" We lasted about two weeks then went back to being friends.

In the seventh grade, I got my second boyfriend—I actually asked him out (this was a big deal). We were sitting in biology class, writing notes back and forth. In about the third note, I asked him to be my boyfriend. I still remember his response. The note read, "If you're joking, it's not funny. If you're not, I'd say 'What the heck, sure.'" Not exactly the response I had hoped for, but close enough. This was the same boy I'd had a crush on in kindergarten so I guess perseverance pays off. This "relationship" lasted until the seventh grade class picnic when I decided that I liked another boy in my class instead. I picked the easy way out and had my friend tell my boyfriend we were breaking up. It was not very emotional since our behavior had never changed toward each other. We were too young to date, and if we kissed, I don't remember it. We never even went to the mall together. The only difference was that we called ourselves a couple. I had similar "boyfriends" in the eighth grade. Nothing serious at all. It was just a way to say I was "going out." It didn't really mean anything, but at the time it seemed really significant.

When I got to high school, little changed. My best friend, Christine, was the person I confided in about my crushes on different guys. We played the same sports, so we'd talk on bus trips to away games. We always sat together in study hall, joking around and writing notes. She had a steady boyfriend and sometimes the three of us went out together. On the weekends, I would usually stay home, find something to occupy my time, or go to watch my brother or sister play basketball games at college. There were parties on the weekends, but that wasn't really my scene. The crowd usually consisted of people who'd already graduated from high school and they would be drinking and all that. I never felt very comfortable at those parties. It wasn't a matter of feeling left out, rather more a choice of how I wanted to spend my time.

Of course, sometimes it bothered me that I didn't have a boyfriend. I filled most of my time with sports—I played basketball and field hockey all four years, and softball my first three years before switching to track—but it wasn't always enough. I wanted to go out on dates. I wished I had someone to dance with at the school dances, someone to take me to semiformals. In retrospect, I'm glad now that I didn't have a boyfriend. Once you get to college, you realize that you have more opportunities to meet guys, and your relationships with them are much more meaningful than in high school, whether or not they become your boyfriends. High school is high school. Sometimes having or not having a boyfriend seems essential, something your whole life depends on. But there's really no reason to worry. When people said, "Just wait until you get to college and there are a lot of tall guys," I would think, "That's two, three years away! I want to meet somebody now!" But you survive; I certainly did. No one looks at me now and thinks there's something wrong with me because I didn't have a boyfriend in high school. Nobody thinks less of me because I didn't have a lot of guys calling me on the phone back then.

Now I can even imagine how hard it must have been for guys. First of all, I was taller than every other person at school. Also, I had braces up until my sophomore year, and an out-of-control hairdo until I was a senior. Looking back, I don't have to wonder why I didn't have a million dates. I remember when

I was in eighth grade my friends and I found this list the boys had made, rating us girls from one to ten—ten, of course, meaning the best looking. These guys were my friends and they rated me a four. I remember saying, "That stinks! Why am I only a four?" Now, looking at pictures of me in the eighth grade, I think the guys were being kind.

Going to UConn was a new experience. I had a lot to adjust to academically, athletically, and socially. I became more open, more likely to behave the way I do when I'm around my family. Overall, when I got to college, I could finally be more myself. I'm naturally a bit of a smartass, and in college people understood where I was coming from. In high school I was more reserved and maybe a little quieter. It was a world apart from the person I was at home.

I must admit that I was quite happy to walk around campus and see men taller than myself. This was new. For the first three years of college, I was interested in different guys and had guys interested in me. My taste varied. I liked guys who were tall and skinny and I liked guys who were shorter but bigger. I was attracted to a guy who ended up being a jerk, and suddenly he wasn't my type anymore. Nothing serious ever resulted. I never had a relationship to write home about. In contrast, my roommate Pam had a serious boyfriend the whole time we were in college. So while I went out every weekend with my teammates, Pam rented a movie and stayed in with her boyfriend. She talked to me about issues that arose in her relationship. I always just listened. I could never give advice because she was experiencing things I had never been through.

Pam was notorious for asking questions like what we would name our kids, how old we would be when we got married, where we would live, and so forth. I usually just smiled and joked that I needed to find a boyfriend before I could answer any of her questions. It was fun to think about stuff like that, but it was nothing more than daydreams. I didn't know what my life was going to be like after graduation, never mind years down the road.

I had many great friends who were guys. Especially during my junior year when my mom was experiencing her battle with cancer, I appreciated the support some of them provided. I didn't tell too many people about what was going on, but those who knew were extremely good listeners.

My last year in college was interesting in a lot of ways. I don't think I changed too much from the person I had been. However, because of the power of the media, people's perceptions of me changed. Not only did more people know who I was, but more people looked at me as a celebrity rather than just a tall woman who played basketball. This became particularly apparent after the season ended and I was in *Sports Illustrated* and on *The Late Show with David Letterman*. I was not comfortable with this attention at all!! I had grown accustomed to signing autographs, but suddenly roses were being sent to my room. Letters were slipped under my door by guys who wanted me to call them back. When I was out with friends, guys gave me their phone numbers. During my senior year guys came up to me all the time in bars, particularly when they had been drinking.

"I know you would never go out on a date with me . . ."

"How do you know I'd never go out on a date with you?"

"Well, because of who you are."

"Who do you *think* I am? " I said to one guy, "Why don't you try? You could always call and see if I call you back."

Even stranger to me, I got masses of mail from men who wanted dates. I even received a few marriage proposals. For some reason, I was particularly attractive to men in prison. (Then again, I guess anyone would be attractive to men in prison.) It was an experience that was completely foreign to me, one that I simply did not relate to, and I answered only a few of the letters. I didn't, of course, accept a single marriage proposal. I wasn't at all interested in meeting someone this way. Four years after high school, I realized that being popular wasn't really all that great. There's nothing worse than telling someone that you aren't interested in him. Instead, I'd beat around the bush, I'd tell jokes. I even had someone tell me he thought I was leading him on because I was being so subtle about the fact that I wasn't interested in him. It got to the point where I didn't return phone calls. I know that wasn't the right thing to do, but after a while I just couldn't handle all the excitement. I was content to be with my friends for my last few weeks in college. I liked being surrounded by people who appreciated what our team accomplished while at the same time treated me no differently than they had the year before.

One of the people who did that most effectively was a football player named Dave DeArmas. I could talk to Dave about almost anything that was going on in my life. He treated me like just another girl on campus. It was refreshing. During the season and the weeks that followed, I couldn't seem to stop myself from developing strong feelings for him. However, our relationship remained solely that of friends. It wasn't because he was 5'10" and would be slightly difficult to dance with; it was because he was involved in a five-year relationship. I understood that and respected it. Perhaps that commitment made my behavior around him more relaxed and easygoing.

I first recognized my feelings for Dave when I was around other men. These men were nice and treated me well, but in the back of my mind I wished I was with Dave. I remember getting a really sweet note from a guy saying he was really interested in me and if I had any interest, would I like to go to a formal with him? He came up to me a week later and introduced himself as the person who wrote the note. I couldn't tell him that I had a boyfriend because I didn't have one. It was awkward and it was just my luck. The first guy in college that I really cared about already cared about someone else. I couldn't be with him and I knew it, but there was nothing I could do to change the way I felt.

Toward the end of the school year, Dave broke up with his girlfriend. He didn't do it for me. He did it for himself. He told me that the relationship was not what he wanted anymore. In all honesty, I can't say I was sorry. We started seeing each other right before school ended. This made tryouts for the National Team in Colorado even more difficult, for not only did I have grueling practice schedules, but, for the first time ever, I had someone back home I missed. When I finally returned to Storrs, I had only been gone for three weeks but it seemed like three months. Dave and I spent the entire summer together. It was the first time in my life I needed someone to feel completely whole. This feeling both scared and invigorated me. It scared me because I knew I would eventually have to leave for Colorado to join the National Team and leave him behind. I was invigorated because I knew I was going to have one of the best summers of my life.

One reason Dave appealed to me so much was that he didn't know a whole lot about basketball. I don't like it when people think I'm just a basketball player. It's no fun when people come up to me and all they want to talk about is basketball. When I'm away from the court, basketball is often the last thing I feel like talking about. From the beginning, Dave and I talked about other things. Plus he came from a great family; his parents were wonderful, and they obviously cared a lot about each other and a lot about him. They're originally from Cuba, so Dave's first language is Spanish; he didn't learn English until he was seven years old. He moved to Maryland from Miami when he was fifteen. Yet he is so adaptable, I don't think of him as a city kid or as a southerner or a Cuban.

I felt very comfortable the first time Dave met my mother. I knew I had chosen a good guy and that my mother would like him. He was the first boy I ever brought home. As expected, my mother liked Dave a lot. I could tell because after about twenty minutes she started teasing him. Dave had passed her test.

Before Dave, I never really told my mom about the boys I was interested in or which guy I liked at the time. In fact, I never really told anyone other than Christine; that was one of the few things that I kept completely to myself. In college, when I did tell my mom about someone I had a crush on, I'd regret it because the next time I talked to her on the phone she'd ask, "Well, how's so-and-so?" and I would have to say, "Oh, he's just a friend," or "I don't want to talk about it." So most of the time I kept quiet. I guess I felt it was a big deal to introduce someone to my parents, even if it was just introducing his name in conversation. Maybe I was afraid these guys wouldn't stand up under their scrutiny. So sometimes I mentioned to my parents that I had been out on a date, but I never really opened up to them about my feelings.

This silence didn't mean that we never talked about relationships in a theoretical sense. My mom talks freely and openly about sex, and she has no problem whatsoever with the subject (probably because it's her job to talk about sex and everything related to it!). She also talks about love and how hard it is and how long it takes to know whether you truly are in love. You can ask her anything and she'll give you a straight answer. My parents never allowed me to feel uncomfortable or think I was asking something stupid. The one rule that they never wavered from, however, was that you don't have sex until after marriage. There were all kinds of reasons for this, complicated and simple, but that was the one fact of life they insisted upon. Once that was understood, everything else they felt and believed about love and marriage and the marriages they wanted all of us to make, fell into place.

Now, if Dave and I are arguing or if he does something I don't understand, I call my parents. I ask Mom questions about what is going on and ask Dad questions about what might be going through Dave's head. I used to think my parents couldn't possibly understand because they dated way back in the sixties. Now I'm amazed at how much they do know and I marvel at the fact that, even though many things have changed since then, many have also stayed the same. And although circumstances and times and values may change, human nature doesn't seem to, or at least not as quickly. When my mother responds to my confusion by telling a story about her own confusion at my age, I'm moved. No longer is she my mom telling me, "No, you will not sleep on the couch in Dave's apartment on your visit to Storrs this weekend. You are coming home. I'm on my way to pick you up." She's saying, "I disapprove, but you must make your own decision." Is it only that I am older now, or has she changed, too?

When it comes to the larger questions I'll have to face in the future about the relationship I'm in, I don't even have to ask to know what my parents' feelings are. When people tell me I am an adult and a grown woman and can make my own decisions, I know they're right and I know my parents would not disagree with them. But I was raised in a certain way and there is only so much I can do about that, grown woman or not. There is enough of my mom's voice and enough of my parents' values inside me that it won't matter how old I am. I know I will always ask myself how I would feel if I had a little sister watching every move *I* made. I wouldn't want her running to mom saying, "But Rebecca did it."

Only time will tell exactly where my relationship with Dave will lead. Only time will tell if these feelings continue. Only time will tell if this is going to be the man who is as loving, respectful, and supportive of me as my father is of my mother.

★ 7 ★

A Gift Called Mom

★ *RUTHANN*

Breast cancer. I never expected to hear that diagnosis. Longevity runs in my family, and, to my knowledge, there is no history of breast cancer. In addition to my own exams, I had faithfully scheduled physical examinations every six months following my fortieth birthday. I had mammograms yearly. Surely, it couldn't happen to me!

I stood naked in front of the mirror. Ready to step into the shower, I was distracted by a shadow stretching across my breast that revealed a lump. Although a recent physical exam had turned up nothing, I was disconcerted. Somewhere at the core of my being, I knew this lump meant trouble.

Within twelve hours of my discovery, I had had a mammogram and was facing my radiologist. She could see nothing unusual in the film. She examined the lump with her hands.

"We can do an ultrasound," she offered.

"How soon?" I pressed.

"This afternoon," she answered. It was Friday, December 3, 1993. Suddenly things began to happen very fast. On Monday morning I received a phone call from my gynecologist.

"The radiologist wants you to see a surgeon." The note of concern in his voice elevated my uneasiness.

"If I were your wife," I asked him, "who would you recommend?" So it was that I found myself in the office of a prominent Hartford surgeon whose self-confidence, kindness, and patience provided the support I so desperately needed in the days that followed.

Dr. Kenneth Kern is a tall, broad-shouldered man who traded in his college football uniform for the green scrubs of the operating room. His hair is sprinkled with enough gray to assure me of his experience. He has a demeanor that is both forthright and comforting.

Dr. Kern's initial examination left him suspicious, but there were additional tests to be done. I would know for certain the following day. His call came in the early evening. Dennis and Jason watched my face intently. They were hopeful. "The lump is malignant," I told them firmly. Tears welled in their eyes. "We'll see the doctor tomorrow." The worst was yet to come.

I was overwhelmed with the enormity of the diagnosis. I wanted to allay the fear I saw in the faces of my son and husband, but I first needed to quiet my own. I replayed in my head the positive messages that I had heard over the years about early detection. I reviewed my own health history. I thought of friends who had survived this diagnosis. Finally, I faced the task of telling relatives and friends.

I called my mother. In disbelief, she asked me to repeat myself.

"I am having surgery on Monday," I said again. Forty questions. I had no answers. "I am having a lumpectomy; we are hopeful that will take care of it." Then Mom asked the obvious question:

"Have you told the girls yet?"

"I'm going to tell them this weekend. I don't want to wait too long because I don't want them to think I keep important things from them. On the other hand, I don't want them to worry needlessly. I'll wait until after the Virginia game to tell Rebecca."

On December 11, the UConn Huskies faced the Virginia Cavaliers. Entering the game with an exhilarating string of victories, the Huskies played their hearts out to stave off a Cavalier run in the second half and defeat their opponents. Rebecca led her team in scoring, rebounding, and blocked shots. She lifted her arms in victory at the end of the game. It should have been a night for celebration.

We waited for Rebecca to complete the postgame session with the team and the interviews with the media. We waited for the signing of autographs requested by patient fans who lingered in Gampel until the players appeared after their showers. We waited until we saw her flushed, happy face as she bounced up the bleachers toward us. I hugged and praised her. I spoke matter-of-factly, "I have something I need to tell you."

Nodding toward the upper bleachers, I suggested we move to a more secluded spot. As we settled into the seats in Section 109, I saw Chris Dailey, the associate head coach, approaching. "You should hear this too, Chris." Chris's presence not only saved me from repeating my story, but it assured me that Rebecca would have support when I left for home. "Listen, Rebecca," I began, "they've discovered a lump in my breast. It's malignant." Alarm. "I am going to have surgery on Monday. They are hoping that by removing the lump, they will be able to get everything." Tears began to flow. "Look, Rebecca," I continued, "the best thing you can do for me is to continue to work hard. I don't want to have to worry about you too. You do what you have to do, and I'll do what I have to do." The ride home from Storrs was bleak. I didn't know how to think about my future.

On Monday, December 13, I arrived at Hartford Hospital for a lumpectomy. Under local anesthesia, I observed the steady hand of my surgeon as he worked skillfully to remove the deadly disease that had invaded my body. I joked with his assistant. I left feeling confident and comfortable. I stopped by the school to assure my colleagues that I was on my way to recovery. That afternoon, Den and I made our way to a game at

Boston College. I wanted my presence at the game to assure my daughter that I felt fine and the surgery had gone well.

On Wednesday, December 15, Den and I trekked into Hartford to once again meet with Dr. Kern. "How are you?" he questioned as he led us to his office. "Well, I don't know, you tell me," I quipped. The flash of pain across his face told me that the news wasn't good. The lump was small but the damage was big. I needed a mastectomy. Dr. Kern was remarkable. He explained in detail what needed to be done and why. He was positive. He gave me both his home and office numbers and encouraged me to call anytime. I clutched the piece of paper bearing those numbers like a child clinging to her security blanket. Later that night, I lay in my husband's arms and wrestled with the mental anguish that would torment me in the months to come.

I arrived at work as usual on Thursday morning, December 16. Surrounded by supportive and caring friends and colleagues, I began to unravel as I told each the news. Some encouraged me to go home, but I knew that being alone with my thoughts was unhealthy. I vacillated between normality and unreasonable fear. Alone in my office, I cried uncontrollably as I watched the normal progression of the day through altered vision. Never again would my life or the way I looked at it be the same. Brenda Pfeiffer, a fellow counselor, quietly offered strength and assistance. Sheri Dorfsman, the school social worker, listened to my fears. Stan Pestka, my principal, allowed me to sift through my thoughts in his office. Kathy Sutton and Elaine Shaw, friends and colleagues, held my hand in prayer. I called my surgeon and blubbered. "This is a disease that can work harder on the mind than the body," he said. How true, how true, how true.

On Friday, December 17, I arrived at Hartford Hospital at 9:00 A.M. An article on Rebecca in the morning paper was tucked under my arm. I planned to savor it while waiting for surgery. I answered questions at admissions. "Do you have a living will?" "Will I need one?" I answered. "That's a great question to ask before surgery," I added. "Great morale booster!" The volunteer who pushed my wheelchair seemed excited that I was Rebecca's mother. As he delivered me to a room, he chatted about the team. Dennis, Jason, and Jason's friend Maura kept me company until it was time to go to the operating room. My last surgery had been a tonsillectomy. I felt alone and frightened as my family disappeared from view.

The young anesthesiologist sat next to me playing twenty questions. I was more concerned about his youth than the questions he was posing. Since when had doctors gone from looking like my father to looking like my son's friends? I established through adroit questioning (Where did you go to school and when did you graduate? How long have you been practicing medicine?) that, in fact, he was responsible and experienced and that I was in good hands. My next stop was the operating room where my surgeon offered encouragement. Fear clutched me. Seeing my panic, my doctor took my hand and held it. As the anesthesia took charge of my body, I surrendered to prayer and the skills of my surgeon.

I awoke in the recovery room to a nurse asking me to wiggle my toes. It was over; the task was done. I waited impatiently to return to my room and see my husband. Sitting next to my bed, Den kissed me and held my hand. Before I could ask, he told me there was one positive lymph node in three that had been examined. The test results on the rest would come later. For the time being, however, I needed to concentrate on recuperating. My spirits were high. I knew that the prayers of many had held me up in crisis. For three days the nurses encouraged me to ask for medication if the pain became unbearable; they told me not to be a martyr. I waited for the pain to come; it never did. I took call after call after call. Flowers arrived nonstop. Thinking the worst was behind me, I looked forward to returning home.

My mother and dozens of flowers awaited when I arrived home on December 20. I felt good. I knew from initial reports that chemotherapy was in order. My first appointment with the oncologist was scheduled for December 22.

★ *REBECCA*

The nurse rubbed alcohol on my arm as she cleansed the skin in preparation to insert the IV needle. She penetrated the vein through which medication would flow so that the doctors could perform the arthroscopic surgery on my knee. It was a simple operation that would take care of my torn cartilage and allow me back on the court in only three weeks.

My body was very relaxed and calm. Like every other time in my life when I needed someone, my mother was at my side. She had held my hand through two surgeries in college and countless visits to the doctor when I was growing up. She was there again only a few feet from where I sat. However, this visit was different. My mom wasn't holding my hand tightly as I squeezed her fingers waiting for the prick like I did when I was younger. She wasn't waiting to wipe the tears from my eyes before they had a chance to fall. Instead, when I glanced over, I saw my mom shedding and wiping her own tears. Without asking, I knew exactly what they were for. Just a year before this simple operation of mine, needed only to put me back on the basketball court, my mother was sitting in a similar chair, with a similar IV in her arm waiting for the chemicals to enter her body to kill the cancer and help her return to a normal healthy life. As I watched her eyes fill up, mine did the same. I immediately turned my head, looked away and hoped and prayed that I would not start crying.

My mom is known in our house for crying at almost anything. She cries when telling stories, listening to songs, reminiscing, even watching television commercials. When we were growing up, Rachel, Jason, and I would just look at each other and roll our eyes whenever we saw our mom have one of these emotional displays. She embarrassed us; she made us uncomfortable when she cried. As we grew older, we just laughed and teased her. It still strikes me funny sometimes how a woman who is so strong in her convictions, beliefs, and actions can be so emotional at the same time.

Amazingly, however, I saw my mom cry the least while she was fighting the cancer. I'm sure she shed buckets of tears, she'd just never let me see them. She was probably feeling the weakest physically during this time than any other point in her life. Emotionally, however, she appeared stronger to me than ever before. I'll never forget her courage the day she told me about the results of her biopsy. She pulled me aside following the game against Virginia my junior year and informed me that a lump was found in her breast and that the lump was malignant. I began to cry and she told me to stop. "Your father isn't a breast man anyway," she said.

Sitting next to me was a woman who just found out she had breast cancer. Here I was, a woman who just played one of the best games of her career and competed in one of her team's biggest victories. It seemed to me that the wrong woman was crying. Then again, you just had to look at who these women were. The woman who was the strength, the comforter, the giver of life, was the mother. The woman who needed strength, comfort, and life, was the daughter. We were filling the roles once again that we had so comfortably accepted the past twenty years. It had to be the scariest thing my mother ever told me. Yet, the same woman who cried with me when I asked her to tell me the truth about Santa Claus displayed only confidence when she told me about her cancer. Just as she had promised me that, even without Santa, Christmas would be the same, my mother was again promising me that everything would turn out just fine. In the same way she made me promise not to tell my brother and father there was no Santa Claus, now she made me promise not to let her news affect my schoolwork or my basketball.

I must admit, the promise about Santa was much easier to keep.

I went to class, practiced hard, and studied as much as my time would allow. Two days after mom told me about the malignancy, she was scheduled to have the lump in her breast removed. It was a Monday and we were to play at Boston College that evening. She told me that if she felt up to it, she would attend. I didn't expect to see her there. I figured that I'd treat the game like a long road trip and just phone the results home after the game ended. The team was doing stretches when I looked up and saw my mother and father take their seats in the stands. Mom looked as if she was coming from just another day at work. She smiled at the other parents, not letting her expression betray the events of her day. I was much less successful at hiding my feelings. A few years before, I would have rolled my eyes if I saw someone on the court with tears in her eyes. That day I didn't care who saw me. It was a day that began a ritual I will take with me for the rest of my career. Now when stretching before games, I check the stands to find my parents. Fortunately, I haven't yet seen an empty seat.

After Boston, we had about two weeks before our next game. Our basketball schedule was structured to allow us time to study for final exams. After my last final, I returned to my room to have my roommate, Pam, tell me I needed to call my father right away. I called home and my dad told me that my mom was in the hospital recovering from a mastectomy. He

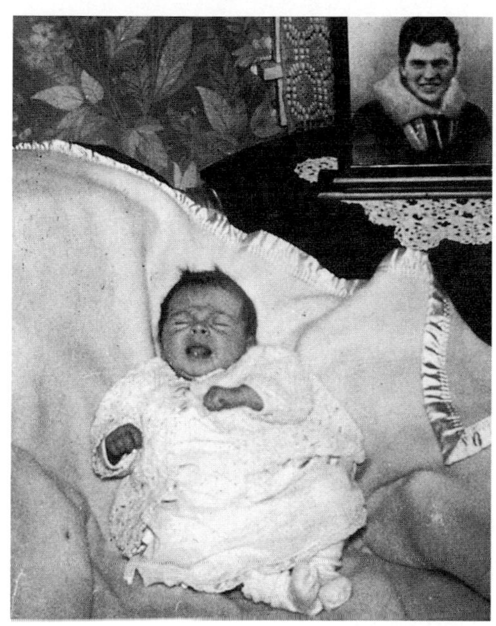

Is anybody listening? (RuthAnn at eight weeks, with a photograph of Jimmy McLaughlin.)

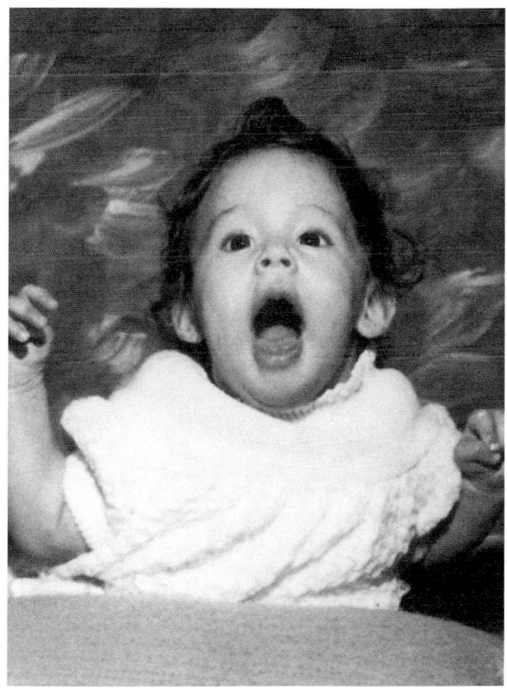

Give me a U, Give me a C, Give me an O-N-N! (Rebecca at three months.)

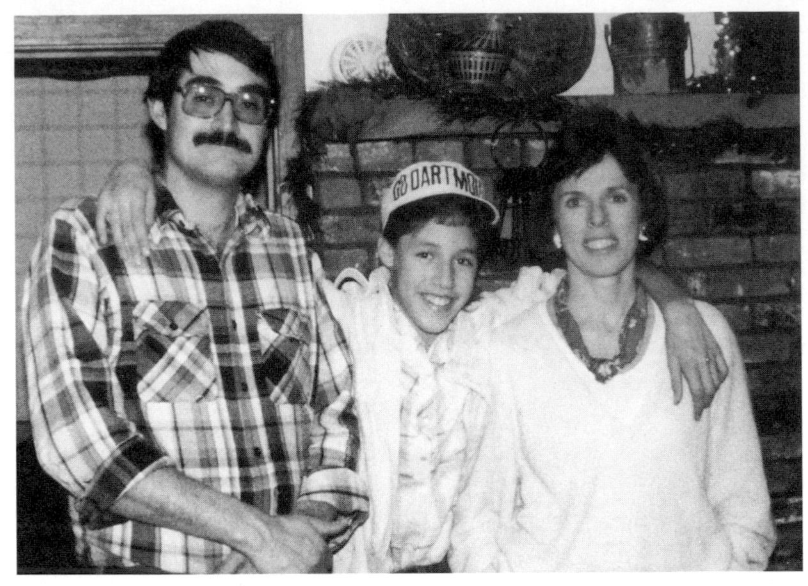

Dennis, the Hat-With-A-Kid-Under-It, and RuthAnn (1986).

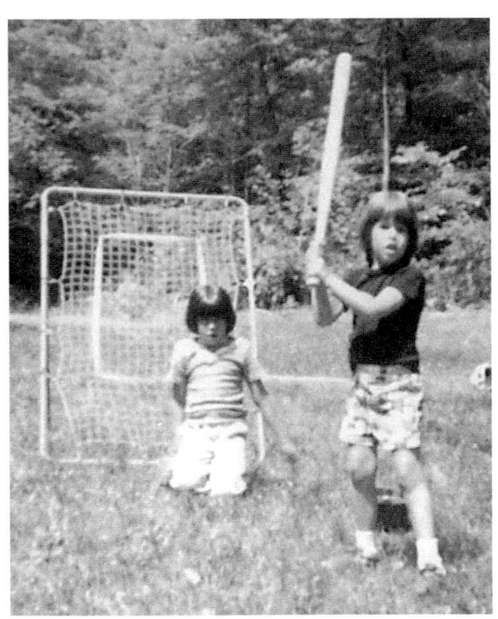

Rachel and Rebecca (foreground) play an after-dinner Wiffle-ball game.

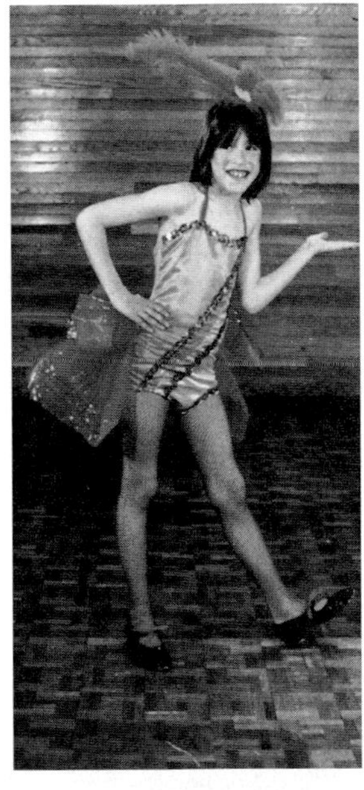

May I show you some fancy footwork? (Rebecca in fishnets, 8 years.)

Rebecca, planning to be the first woman to play for the Boston Celtics.

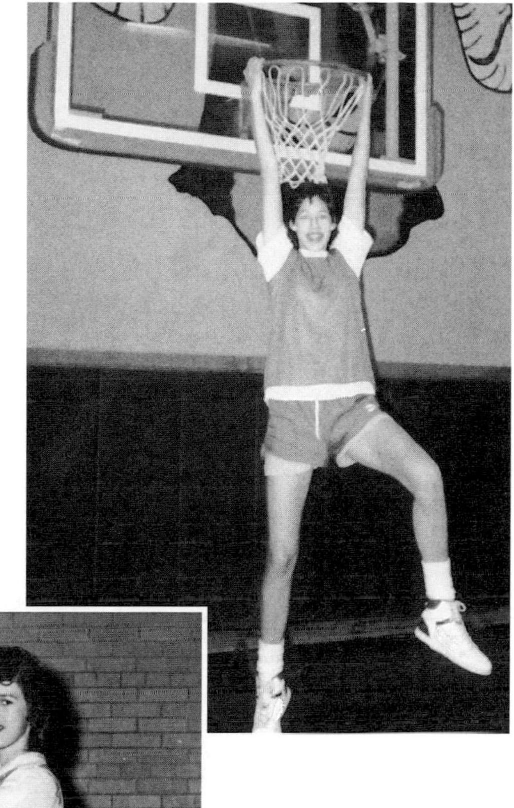

RuthAnn, a.k.a. Turnpike ("you can go for miles without a curve in sight."), Medfield High School Basketball Team, 1961.

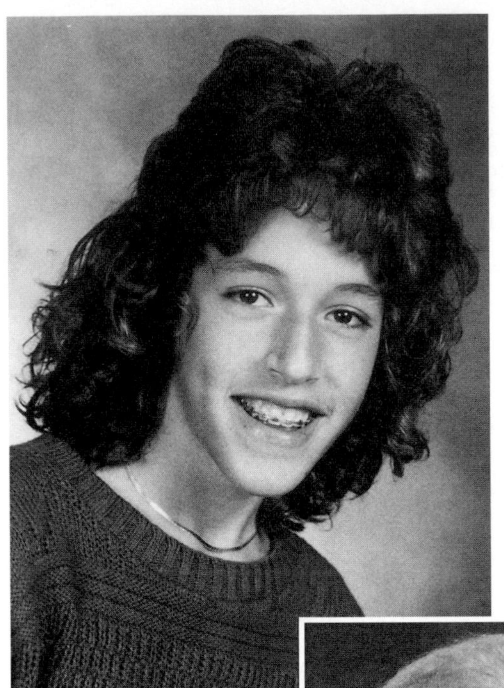

Today, when Rebecca looks in horror at her high school pictures and asks me why I didn't say anything about her hairstyle, I respond in the same way my mom did when I asked her: "I tried to tell you but you wouldn't listen!"

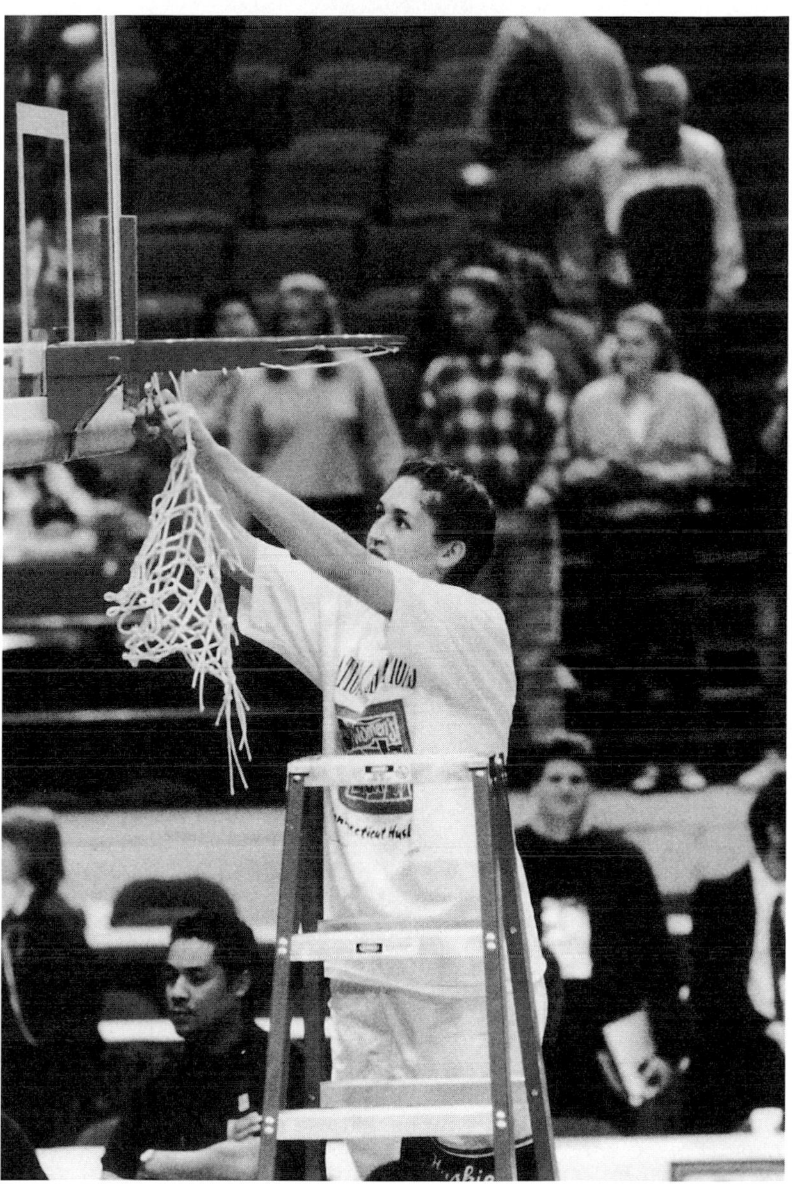

The perfect end to a perfect season. Rebecca cuts the net after the UConn women win the national championship in Minneapolis.
(University of Connecticut Division of Athletics/Bob Stowell, Photographer.)

Pam Webber and Rebecca, roommates and teammates for four years, enjoy a victory. (Reprinted with permission of *The Hartford Courant*/ Shana Sourek Mei.)

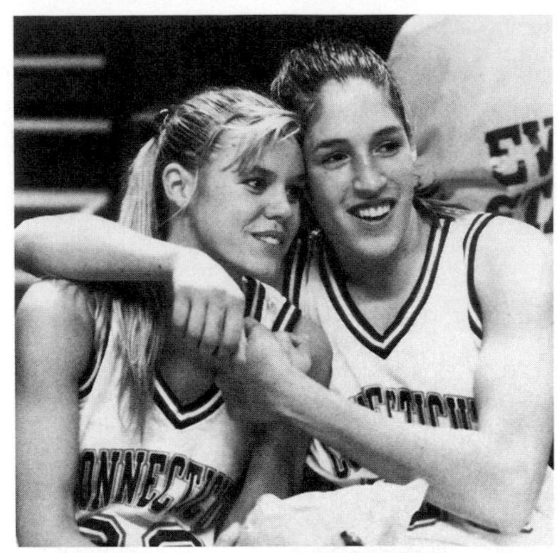

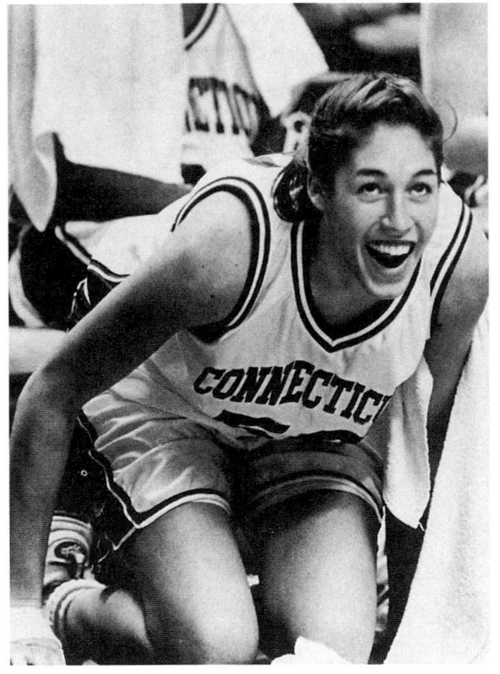

Rebecca breaks into a grin as UConn upsets the unbeaten Tennessee Volunteers on January 14, 1995 and is elevated to #1 in the polls. (Photo © 1995 by Carl E. Hartdegen.)

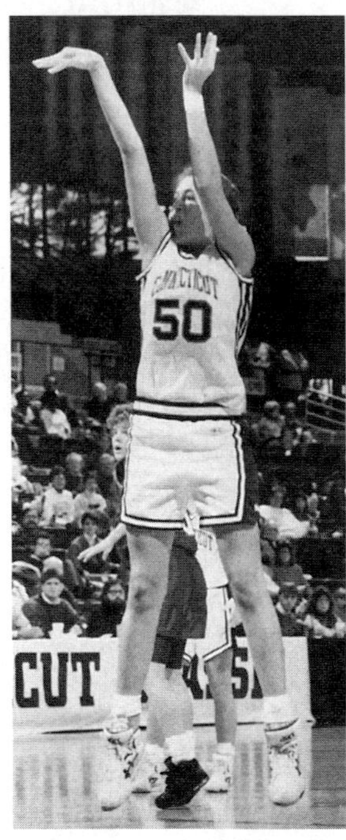

Gampel Pavilion, home sweet home. (University of Connecticut Division of Athletics/Bob Stowell, Photographer.)

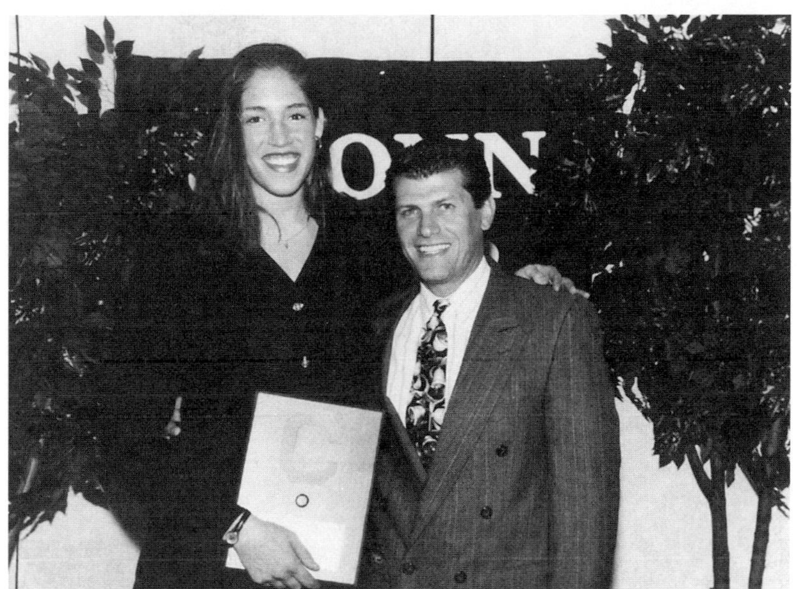

With Coach Auriemma. In my heart I'll always be a Husky! (University of Connecticut Division of Athletics/Bob Stowell, Photographer.)

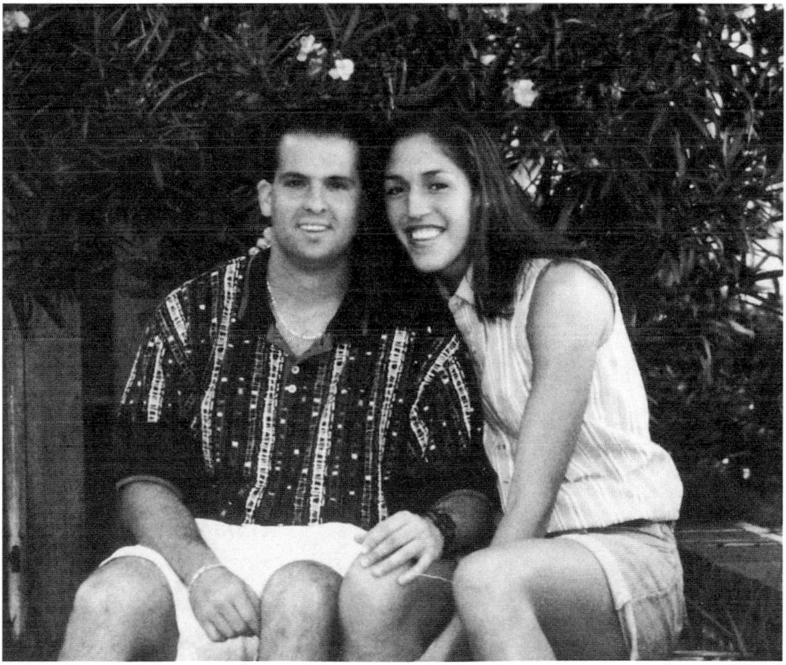

The other man in my life, Dave. (Photo by Rachel Lobo.)

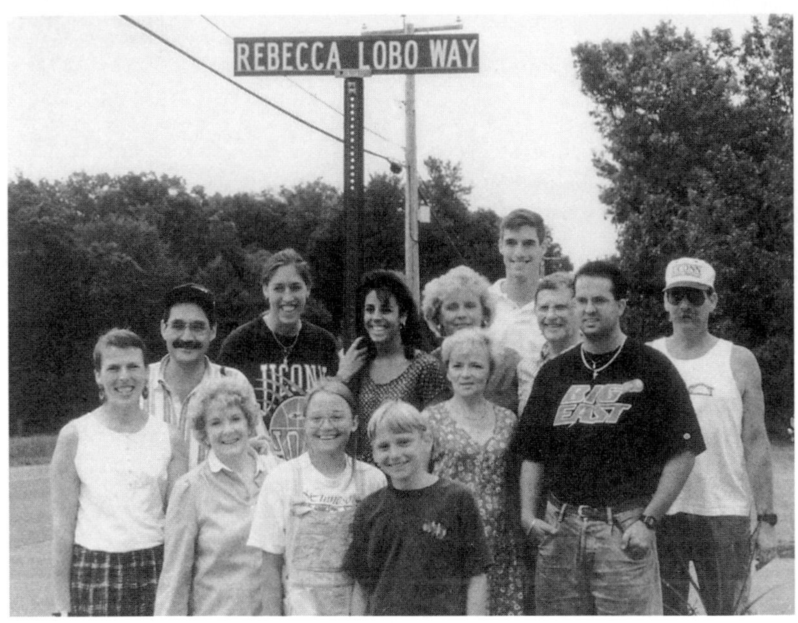

From left, clockwise: RuthAnn, Dennis, Rebecca, Rachel, Jason, and an assortment of grandparents, aunts, uncles, and cousins join the celebration as Southwick declares Rebecca Lobo Day (August 12, 1995) and names a street in Rebecca's honor. (Photo by David Pierce.)

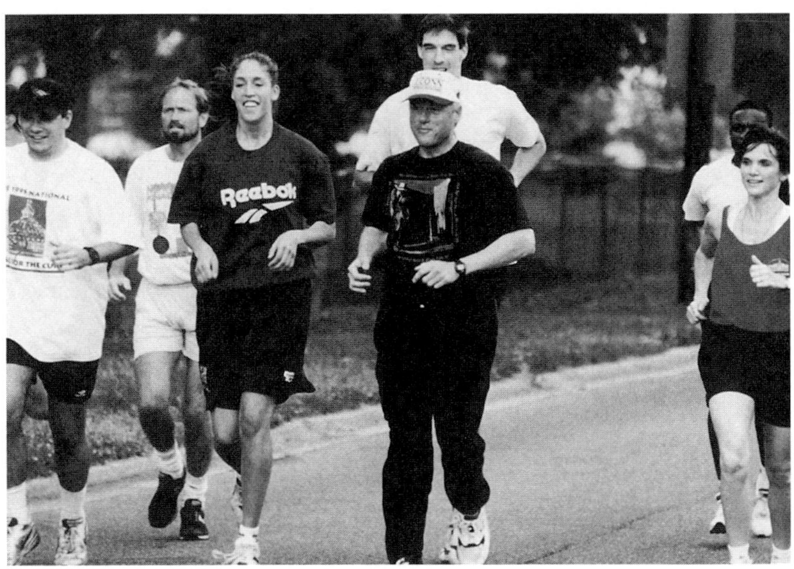

Run, women, run! Official White House photo, June 21, 1995.

also informed me that she was going to have to undergo chemotherapy. Up to this point I believed that chemo would be unnecessary. I thought that the lumpectomy was going to be sufficient. Unfortunately, I was very wrong.

My mother had been in the hospital for two days, having pressured my father not to tell me until my finals were over—she was afraid I would be distracted. Even when facing one of the scariest times in her life, my mother was worried about her children! I hung up the phone, sat on the couch, and cried and cried. In between sobs and tears I told Pam what my father had told me. I felt so helpless. I wanted to be able to do something to help my mom but knew that my hands were tied. I left the room and walked across campus to St. Thomas Aquinas, the Catholic church on campus. I entered and found myself alone. I prayed for almost an hour. I believed God would listen. I simply knew that this was the only place where I could feel better or even have a chance to do some good for my mom.

After I completed my finals and the fall semester ended, my parents brought me home for what amounted to a three-day Christmas break. It was the longest holiday since I entered UConn. The day I arrived home, my mother and father were going to meet with the oncologist for the first time. I went with them. On the ride over, as my mom read her Bible, I realized she was scared. It was the first time I ever actually saw her scared for herself. She was worried about the number of lymph nodes in which cancer had been found. Apparently, anything over ten was considered dangerous, because the nodes indicated how far the cancer had spread.

I'll never forget that day, sitting in the oncologist's office. She talked about the cancer, about treatments, and about the lymph nodes. She said they found cancer in twenty-eight of them. TWENTY-EIGHT. That number escaped from her lips and entered my heart like a dagger. I could do nothing to prevent the tears from falling in a continuous downpour. I could only wipe them away again and again. I remember looking at my father and seeing his eyes fill up, too. I wanted to run out of the room so badly, as if the doctor's words wouldn't be true if I could leave them in the office. Then I looked at my mom. She just sat there with her pad and pen on her lap, listening. She didn't have a tear in her eye. She simply asked the doctor to repeat the different available treatments so she could write them down. Then she asked me if I was all right. Now I see that it was probably easier to imagine how I was feeling and calm my fears than to turn and face her own. At the time, however, it seemed unreal that she could spare a thought for me. The look on her face told me that in no uncertain terms, everything was going to be okay.

No one spoke a word on the drive home. I simply prayed to God to heal my mother. I wished that I could return to the days when Mom and Dad's biggest Christmas-time worry was getting the presents wrapped without the kids seeing them. This Christmas, I didn't care if I received a single gift. I prayed that there would be another Christmas where I could have the chance to pick out a gift for my mom. Once again I cried because there was no Santa. If only there was, I thought, I could go sit on his lap and ask him to bring a miracle cure for my mom.

When we returned home, my mother explained to my brother and sister what the oncologist said. She used the most sugar-coated terms possible. If I had heard only mom's version, and not the doctor's, it would seem like everything was basically fine. Instead of looking to her kids for support, my mother asked us to lean on her. It was as if the only thing keeping her up was belief in God, her husband, and the need to protect her children from their worst fears. I never saw her falter. She did everything she could to make sure her kids saw only the power of her faith, her love, and her courage. This power became part of us all. It is still with us.

★ *RUTHANN*

We had expected a routine visit. Young and freshly scrubbed, Dr. Stacey Nerenstone entered the room wearing a mid-calf length skirt and soft suede boots. Her white lab coat covered her shirt. Long, straight hair fell gently over her shoulders. She seated herself across from me and held my records in her hand. She began to talk about treatment. The tests were back. I already knew there were lymph nodes involved.

"How many?" I asked. To be honest I knew very little about breast cancer. I did know that lymph node involvement in any cancer diagnosis isn't good. I had been hearing about women with six, seven, ten affected lymph nodes. Not good, they said. Dr. Nerenstone replied stoically. "Twenty-eight."

She continued. I made eye contact. I feigned attention. She thought I was listening, but I never heard another word. Fear had gripped the back of my neck and raced its icy fingers over every cell in my body. As the doctor's voice provided a monotone backdrop, I succumbed to a terror I had never known before. I caught a glimpse of my husband and child who were both overcome with the magnitude of the doctor's words. Tears rolled quietly down their cheeks. I wanted to escape my body, my mind! I wanted to erase my fear and panic! I could not believe this was happening to me.

At some point during that visit I collected myself. Looking squarely at the oncologist, I said flatly,

"I haven't heard a thing you've said since you told me about the lymph nodes. Let's go over my options for treatment again." I tried to listen the second time and jotted down notes. I left the office in a state of despair.

"I can't imagine why she would want to do this for a living," Rebecca blurted out on the way home.

"Because she wants to save lives," I replied dryly.

When we arrived home, my mind was racing. Jason and Rachel were waiting for us. I explained as best I could the recommendations of the oncologist. Rachel peppered me with dozens of questions until I finally exploded.

"Stop asking me all these questions!" I snapped at her. "I don't have the answers." Bursting into tears, she ran upstairs. She was desperate for assurance that everything would be all right. So was I.

Our Christmas tree stood half-decorated in the living room. There were no Christmas cookies or gingerbread men this year. Decorations remained in boxes. I sank into a chair in the living room completely wretched. I wondered if this were to be my last Christmas celebration.

The next day, December 23, I took Rebecca for some last-minute shopping. When we returned, the driveway was full of cars. My spirits brightened. Kathy Sutton was busily preparing dinner in the kitchen. A teacher from an elementary school in Granby was dropping off some goodies. Donny Drzyzga, a friend of Rachel's, and his mom had dropped by to check in. My counter was laden with Christmas cookies from teachers at Granby High School. I was touched by the goodness and generosity of people who found time for our family during this busy time of year.

I returned to work immediately following Christmas break, seeking the comfort that comes from routine and familiar faces. People conveyed their support in a variety of ways; some asked about my health, some sent me funny cards, some made dinners, some prayed with me, some expressed their concern by saying nothing at all. Each person had his or her own way of helping me feel needed and loved.

Visits to the surgeon and oncologist became more pressing as the time for treatment drew closer. They discussed reconstructive surgery. I wasn't interested. In a way I was surprised by my response. I found myself walking past Victoria's Secret, mournfully eycing the lacy lingerie. "I'll never be able to shop there again," I thought with sadness. "Who are you kidding?" I caught myself, "You never even shopped there in the first place!" In the big picture the loss of a breast was insignificant.

The doctors insisted that I needed as much chemotherapy as I could get. They presented options. I was asked to make decisions for which I had no expertise. I wanted guarantees. There were none. They encouraged second opinions. I traveled to Boston. In the waiting room I watched a young mother clutch her toddler to her breast before turning the child over for blood work. How does a mother explain to a little one she loves the ordeal of disease and treatment? Drawing on the intimacy of that mother and child, I chastised myself for self-pity. I returned home assured that treatment offered in Hartford was equal to the best in the country. I was ready to begin.

The treatment I chose entailed four massive treatments of chemotherapy every three weeks starting at the end of January. I arranged my treatments around the UConn women's basketball schedule. I was determined not to miss a game.

The first treatment fell on Martin Luther King's birthday. We drove to the Harry and Helen Gray Cancer Clinic at Hartford Hospital. Judy Grasso, the nurse who was my support during treatments, waited to escort me to a room filled with the tools of the trade. Her quiet voice and pleasant manner were soothing. Judy Kulko, the administrative nurse whose ear I bent over the next six months, offered warmth and encouragement. Den and I chatted. We read. I sat in the recliner and the IV needle was inserted into my arm. The treatment was underway.

Snow began to fall steadily outside the window. As the powerful drugs made their way into my bloodstream, I drifted off into sleep. At five o'clock, professing to feel just fine, I climbed into the car and headed for home. The snow was still falling and its accumulation promised a long and tortuous ride home. Dennis drove at a snail's pace and decided to leave the highway for safer passage on back roads. The forty-minute trip stretched into an hour plus. I don't remember; I slept all the way home.

I returned to work two days later feeling quite comfortable. There was a hint of nausea, nothing I couldn't handle. If that was the worst of it, I thought, I would be okay. Sheri accompanied me to the second treatment. We took word games with us. As the chemicals entered my body, I found it difficult to see the letters and to think creatively. I teased my friend, accusing her of taking advantage of my weakened condition. I returned to work three days later but with less ease than the first time. Food held little appeal and waves of nausea interrupted my routine. Nancy Oates, our guidance office secretary, mother-henned me. The administration adjusted my workload, and a coworker absorbed some of my responsibilities. My eighth-grade guidance aides, Emily Hoffman, Jennifer Pomponi, and Megan Gremelspacher, manned my office when I arrived late. I laughingly accused them of vying for my job but in truth I was touched beyond words by their reliability and trustworthiness.

Rebecca's basketball games took on new meaning for me. Not only were they benchmarks around which I scheduled my treatments, they were something to look forward to. I was determined not to worry my daughter by my absence at a game. The UConn basketball family reached out in countless ways of support. Coach Auriemma called me at home and at work to see how I was doing. He and Coach Dailey brainstormed for locations in Gampel where I could watch the games free from the risk of germs if my blood count dropped too low. Flowers and notes arrived from the players, their parents, and the athletic department. I knew my daughter was surrounded by good people.

As if on cue, my hair began to fall out in handfuls by the sixth week. I had decided to christen my wig on the first day of school following February vacation. In my naïveté I hoped that the week-long break would dull the students' sensitivity to my new hairdo. I would have been just as discreet if I had worn a coonskin cap! As always, I entered the building through the rear entrance, which leads into the sixth-grade wing. Through the door window, I saw the students busily milling about in preparation for homeroom. Suddenly, I too was an adolescent, gripped with the fear of being noticed. I wanted to turn and run. I contemplated other entries. Finally, I braced myself and muttered, "Just do it, RuthAnn. Just dig deep and do it." I opened the door and stepped inside. I spotted a few quizzical looks as I held my head high and focused on my destination. One boy beamed, "I like your hair, Mrs. Lobo." Give that kid a kiss!

Each time I ventured into new territory with my wig, I worried about exposure, ridicule, and rejection. The first time I wore it to Gampel Pavilion, I feared a million inquiries about my new appearance. It didn't happen. Rebecca spotted me during warm-ups and masked her dismay with a heart-warming smile. There were some awkward moments as well. Late in the season, a well-intentioned woman approached me after one of the games to tell me how much she liked my new hairstyle.

"Thank you," I said.

"I can't get over how full it is," she continued, "It's quite flattering." I smiled. "Can you give me the name of your hairdresser?" she persisted.

"The truth is," I responded, "I'm undergoing medical treatment, and I'm wearing a wig!" Did she make a hasty retreat!

I approached my third treatment with less than my usual enthusiasm. I had been down-hearted, and tears welled up as Dr. Nerenstone entered my room.

"All week," I confessed, "I've been telling myself I'm dying." Dr. Nerenstone looked at me and laughed. It was the best sound in the world.

"You're not dying," she admonished. "You're fighting."

* * * *

On the following Thursday, Barbara Cohen and I accompanied six students to a talk show in New York. As Title IX compliance coordinators in Granby, our role is to see that every employee at school understands the law regarding equity and sexual harassment. In response to a show on harassment, Barbara wrote a letter that earned us an invitation to appear with our students in the audience and to possibly share our perspective.

We traveled to New York in style, in a stretch limousine. We sat through two tapings of the show, had lunch in a trendy New York restaurant, and returned to our limo for the two-hour ride home. Suddenly my body announced I had demanded too much of it. I was overcome with waves of discomfort as we made our way back toward Connecticut. "Please God," I prayed, "don't let me throw up in front of my students." When we arrived at school, I hurried to my car and guided myself the short distance home. I walked into the house and burst into tears. Den looked at me in alarm. "I just overdid it," I said as I made a mad dash for the bathroom.

Basketball kept me going. I read voraciously all the articles about the team. I counted the days between games. I talked about nothing else. After treatments, I'd rest on the couch watching videos of games. When the chemotherapy resulted in my blood count dropping, the nurses suggested I avoid crowds to guarantee less chance of infection. Dr. Nerenstone knew better.

"Just don't kiss anybody," she smiled. One Saturday I felt particularly nauseous. Nothing helped. I finally reached the doctor on call.

"What medications are you taking?" he questioned. After hearing my prescriptions, he responded, "Well, you've already got all the big guns. Can you go to bed and rest for the day?"

"Sure," I replied out loud. "Until three," I said to myself. Rebecca had a game that afternoon and I intended to be there.

The rides to the game often found me muddled in my deepest, darkest thoughts. Unlike the previous two years when my greatest anxiety while driving to Gampel was the outcome of the night's game, I thought about how quickly my life had changed. Suddenly my mind was transfixed on the number of games I would live to see. I pushed thoughts of death to the outer reaches of my thinking, but in amoebalike fashion they oozed back into my consciousness to attack my peace of mind. We were given a parking space near Gampel Pavilion to minimize my walking distance; I would have preferred good health and the walk.

With a new awareness, I treasured the sights and sounds of the pavilion. The enthusiasm of the crowd, the smell of the popcorn, the sparkle of the cheerleaders, and the zeal of the pep band were crisp and clear. I inhaled the pure sportsmanship and athleticism of the game. It was, after all, only a game. Young women testing their skills in a game they loved, surrounded by an arena of fans who loved them in return. In the middle of it all, I would momentarily detach myself and wonder if I would be there the following year to again be a part of it and to see Rebecca complete her college career.

Our decision to keep my surgery and treatment private was in deference to all of us, but especially Rebecca, who might be bombarded with queries about my health. Neither Den nor I wanted anything to detract from the hard work and success that was being achieved by Rebecca and her teammates. But at the end of the season it came out. When Rebecca accepted her awards for the Big East Player of the Year at a banquet in a Hartford hotel ballroom, her cheerful gratitude suddenly collapsed. After thanking God, her teammates and coaches, her voice began to falter. She said, "This is for my mother. She has been the real competitor this year, and this is for her." Within minutes, the telephone at home began to ring.

I had somehow expected the interest in my health to subside during the long break between the 1994 and 1995 seasons. It didn't happen. No sooner had the 1995 season begun, when the request for television, newspaper, and magazine interviews overwhelmed us. The initial questions varied but ultimately turned toward my battle with breast cancer. The lump in my throat would rise, my voice would become hoarse and I would begin to blubber. Of course, it was always those moments that made it to the TV screen. I told Dennis, "People watching these TV programs must think, 'What's the matter with that woman; she's always crying.'" We were eager to put the whole episode behind us and move ahead.

I discovered, however, that people in a variety of circumstances, and especially those dealing with cancer, were, for whatever reason, identifying with us. I was taken aback by the number of people who either wrote or stopped by in person to share a tiny morsel of their lives. It always started the same way. A person, usually a woman, would engage me in conversation about Rebecca, the team, or the game of the moment. Then, dropping her voice, she would draw closer. "We have something in common," she'd whisper, at which point I would hear of a trial and/or triumph with breast cancer. It was shocking how many people had suffered. At first I was troubled because I had nothing to offer in return. It was humbling to be the recipient of so much personal and heart-rending disclosure. After a time, I stopped asking why. If someone found solace in talking to me, I made myself available to listen. It was an honor.

★ *REBECCA*

It was a Christmas I'll never forget, although I wish that I could. It's very difficult to get excited about a holiday that celebrates new life when it seems like something is working to take life away. I went shopping on the 23rd. It was just about the only time in my life I left something until the last minute. I bought the standard gifts for everyone except for my mom. On the night before Christmas Eve, I sat at the kitchen table and started to write a poem. It ended up being my gift to her.

When I look in the mirror
Asking "What do I see?"
Is it a reflection of you
Or a reflection of me

When I read the words
Written before me high and low
I learn something new
That you already know

When I walk with a shadow
Casting outlines of me
I have to look twice
Easily you it could be

When I think to myself
Who I'll be, what I'll do
I hope and I pray
I'll be something like you

I had this poem put onto a picture of myself playing basketball that was taken during our game against Virginia. I put the picture in a mirror frame and entitled it "Reflections." I felt, and still feel, that I'll be pretty lucky if there are reflections of my mom in me.

Of course, I've only come to feel that way since I've gotten older. There were countless times when I was younger that I told my mom I was going to treat my kids totally differently from the way she treated me. When I was a teenager I promised myself that I would never embarrass my daughter the way my mother embarrassed me. I would not give my kid a bedtime and her curfew would be just as late as everyone else's. Whenever I announced these plans to Mom, she always used the same comeback. She said, " I hope your daughter acts just like you. I hope she turns out just like you."

Looking ahead, I know that I am going to embarrass my daughter. I'll give her a bedtime and a curfew earlier than her friends'. I hope I treat her exactly the way my mom treated me. And I must admit that I won't be too disappointed if she acts a little bit like I did. If she ever tells me that I'm a bad mom, I'll say, "I hope your daughter acts just like you. I hope she turns out just like you." And if I do even half as good a job raising her as my mom did me, it won't be a bad cycle to perpetuate.

However, I wouldn't like to see the chapter of my mother's life with breast cancer repeated in my own. Granted, her illness helped me grow up a lot and put things into a clear perspective. The threat of losing her helped me fully appreciate this woman who offers so much. Our daughters should not have to worry about losing one of the most precious gifts they have in their lives before they are fully women themselves. To every young girl arguing with her mother about clothes or boys or curfews, I would like to pass on what I've learned about this gift. A gift that continually teaches and gives and loves. A gift that wants nothing in return. A gift I proudly call "Mom."

✶ 8 ✶

School Days, School Days, Dear Old Golden Rule Days

✶ *RUTHANN*

Two school buses, owned and operated by the Newell Taxi Service, were sufficient transport for my entire high school. I graduated from Medfield High in 1961, a stately edifice that looked across playing fields to the flat-roofed building, affectionately called "Fort Apache," where I had attended elementary school and junior high. The Nebo Knockouts and the Harding Hard Hitters, makeshift football and baseball teams from opposite ends of town, played their hearts out on these playing fields. There were no coaches running organized drills, no parents yelling deprecating comments at their kids or the referees; it was just a bunch of kids getting together to play games they loved. There my friends and I etched hopscotch grids in the dirt, jumped rope, shot marbles, and played Red Rover, Red Rover.

Within the walls of "Fort Apache," I discovered the joys of reading, suffered embarrassing moments, and accumulated friendships and skills for a lifetime. Mrs. Brennan, my fourth grade teacher, read to us each day and unveiled worlds of fantasy and wonder. I was first introduced to Tom Sawyer and Becky Thatcher in her classroom. It was also where I choked back tears when the spider died in *Charlotte's Web,* an embarrassing display I repeated when, as a teacher, I read that story to a fourth grade class.

Over the years I learned to make models of volcanoes, relief maps, and papier maché animals. Skills for a lifetime. I represented my grade in the school spelling bee and was eliminated for misspelling the word *development.* I crafted stories to read out loud to my classmates. I learned not to hang upside down on the jungle gym if I was wearing underwear with a hole in it. I also experienced the humiliation of being singled out and ridiculed by a teacher.

It was in second grade and I was a chatterbox in the first degree. I spent more than a few hours standing in the corner for talking "out of turn." One day my teacher, who was creative in her punishments, pinned a large sign to me that said, "I am a bad girl." I was six years old. I cried silently as I stood before my classmates in disgrace. Several years later, when that same teacher fell ill and was confined to a wheelchair, my child's mind figured that God was punishing her for being so mean.

I sat in classrooms where student misbehavior was confined to note passing, gum chewing, and an occasional prank. On one occasion a Playboy centerfold was attached to the map of the world, waiting to be discovered by the elderly and eccentric history teacher. She ripped the picture down in a fury and summoned the principal to reprimand the offenders. Once my algebra teacher, Mr. Morris, dashed out of our second-floor classroom to chastise several upper-class boys for cursing beneath our open window. At the time, all of this seemed like high drama.

The teacher who influenced me most was Mrs. Pederzini. Her Latin and English classes instilled in me the love of Shakespeare, Latin roots, and writing. Without raising her voice, she maintained discipline and decorum while challenging us to work hard and achieve our best. I have given much thought over the years to Mrs. Pederzini's quiet ability to earn our respect, hold our attention, and inspire our learning. I have never been able to pinpoint any specific technique; her mere presence in the classroom was sufficient to keep the behavior of her students in check. In my four years, she spoke to me only once for talking (I was still a chatterbox). I was mortified to think I had offended this wonderful lady. She also knew me better than I thought. Years after graduation, I stopped by to tell her how much she had influenced my life. She looked me squarely in the eye and said, "RuthAnn, you would go and go and go, and then you'd be out a day to rest and catch up!"

My mother, who had left school impulsively after a disagreement with a teacher, stressed the importance of education. Although I was a good student, I was sometimes frustrated by my mother's expectations. If I received three As and two Bs on my report card, I pointed with pride to the three As. Mom focused on the Bs. "If you can get As in three subjects," she reasoned, "you should be able to get As in the other two."

As our children embarked on their school careers, lunch boxes in hand, we encouraged them to do their best. Schoolwork was a priority; sports and clubs were allowed only when schoolwork was done. No televisions, telephones, or video games were permitted in the kids' bedrooms because such gadgets isolate kids from the rest of their family. Until high school all homework was done at the kitchen table. Den was better at helping than I was. The kids complained that I insisted on teaching them the entire lesson when all they wanted to know was "how to do this one little thing."

Jason, affable and even-tempered by nature, loved school from the beginning. His first grade teacher was baffled by how to handle his Show and Tell contributions. At each opportunity to share, Jason volunteered to sing. Standing in front of the class, he created songs that went on and on and on. My only visit to the school on disciplinary issues came when, in middle school, he decided to test the patience of his science teacher. Another chatterbox, Jason spent more time talking than working with his lab partner.

Rachel was the child I pictured as the quiet Lobo in school. That image was shattered when her friend revealed that, while the teacher was out of the classroom, my middle child had led the class in a McDonald's jingle while standing on top of her desk. Unlike her brother and sister, she rebelled at my inquiries about her assignments and did them in bed by flashlight or not at all. When she was in the eighth grade, I was notified that her schoolwork was slipping and so too were her grades. I initiated a short-term accountability system with her teachers in order to monitor her work. Rachel was miffed.

"You said you didn't care about my grades as long as I did my best," she argued.

"Are you doing your best?" I asked. "Can you honestly tell me that all of your work is done? Are you studying each night? Are you giving this your best effort?" Her eyes dropped to the floor.

"No," she mumbled. After six weeks of close supervision, she was back on track and the monitoring system ended.

Rebecca was an extremely conscientious student. Her motivation and self-discipline were evident from the beginning of her school career. She set high standards for herself and became disgruntled if she failed to meet them. She loved to read and knew how to budget her time. Impatience with herself and others brought me to school on several occasions. Her fourth grade teacher reported that Rebecca showed little tolerance for students who didn't grasp concepts quickly and complained when they couldn't find the answer that was already hers. "How can you not get that? It's so *easy*," she blurted out in class. The combined efforts of school and home helped Rebecca to become more sensitive to those around her.

If Rebecca was hard on others, she was even harder on herself. During her middle school years, she threw a fit in the middle of a field hockey game by throwing her stick on the ground after she had been called for a foul. This act of poor sportsmanship was felt by many, including me, to be an affront to the official. When I later asked her about it, Rebecca was surprised to hear how I viewed it. "I wasn't mad at the official, Mom," she explained, "I was mad at myself for committing the foul!" In eighth grade, she insisted on dropping band because the only B on her report card had been in that subject. Alarmed at the importance she was assigning to A's, I told her that I would rather see more B's on her second quarter report card. Band stayed.

It is essential that children understand that mistakes are part of life and are not to be used to evaluate our inner goodness. Children have a tendency to read a grade on a report card as an assessment of their character, even without encouragement from their parents to do so. They beat themselves up verbally and emotionally if they don't do well, they become smug if they do. They forget that a grade is only one indication of how well a small bit of information is mastered in a short period of time. A bad grade can indicate poor study habits or time mismanagement, but little else. And it certainly won't reveal the kind and tender heart. Likewise, a flubbed shot on the basketball court is not the end of the world. The key is to learn, to adjust, and improve from those mistakes. (Like it was that easy!)

Throughout their total of thirty-six years of school, my children accumulated a wealth of skills and experiences that they still recount with warmth and affection. Talk around our dinner table not only focused on the lessons of the day but on interesting science experiments, math challenges, and which teachers had a fashion sense, which didn't. There was only one year out of thirty-six that we remember as the "year from hell."

Rebecca had started one elementary school year on a sour note by being falsely accused in front of the class for cheating on a test. My efforts to resolve the tension between her and this teacher were apparently interpreted as my lack of confidence in the teacher's ability and I succeeded only in alienating her. As the year progressed, further conflicts arose and because I didn't seem to be able to help matters, Rebecca and I agreed that she would resolve them herself. My one condition was that she would tell me of every incident. So I heard of how Rebecca was scolded for not wearing her coat out to recess, how she was reprimanded for peeling contact paper from a table in the classroom, how she was told to mouth the words to a holiday song because her voice was so awful (she refuses to sing to this day), and yes, how she was called a tomboy and berated for wearing pants to school instead of dresses. For me, the last straw fell when she was "punished for being punished" in the cafeteria. Rebecca had joined two classmates in dumping salad and dessert onto another student's pizza at his encouragement. The kids thought it a great joke; the teacher on lunch duty did not. The kids were sent to the office where they sat "in suspension" for part of the afternoon. Upon returning to class, Rebecca was told that she was "spoiled and a brat," and that she had brought disgrace to her classroom by being sent to the office. Her recesses were suspended for the upcoming month.

I listened to my daughter's tale of woe when she arrived home. I was incensed. Although I was not happy with Rebecca's being such a twit in the cafeteria, I was satisfied that she had been adequately punished by the teacher on duty. I was furious that her classroom teacher had not only chosen to impose additional consequences but had once again insulted and belittled her in front of the class.

"I'm going to school to discuss this," I announced, grabbing my bag and car keys. Rebecca's eyes widened in horror and she began to tremble.

"You promised if I told you what was bothering me, you'd let me handle it," she wailed. "You'll only make it worse for the rest of the year."

I watched as my child began to sob and shake uncontrollably. I looked at Dennis. We were both dumbfounded by the magnitude of Rebecca's reaction. Dennis, who normally left the trials and tribulations of the elementary school to me, and who is unusually mild mannered, had a dark expression on his face.

"Get her out of that classroom," he uttered.

As educators, both Dennis and I turned deaf ears on little grumblings that occasionally came home from school. We knew there were two sides to every story. Over the years we were too familiar with the complaints and excuses of students who didn't do homework, couldn't budget time, or wouldn't stop talking. We had seen parents who deprived their children of opportunities to mature by bailing them out of every uncomfortable situation that came along. As Rebecca sobbed hysterically that afternoon in our kitchen, however, we knew that we had to intervene. Jumping in my car, I angrily drove to the school. Luckily, everyone had left. Over the weekend, I weighed my biases as a teacher and parent. On Monday I consulted my own building principal and assistant principal. Confident in my position, I requested a meeting with the teacher. I hoped to affect some change in the classroom, but my efforts were fruitless. Even though I'd tried to avoid it, Rebecca was eventually removed from the classroom.

I learned from that episode that it is frequently the unpleasant incident that is uppermost in our minds when asked to recall our educational experiences. When the "year from hell" invades my memory and conversation, I neutralize my frustration by remembering the many good and productive years my children enjoyed in the public school system: Mrs. Jones, the tender fourth grade teacher who helped Rebecca understand that not everyone grasps a lesson right away; Coach Vincent, who sacrificed much of his own personal time to talk to recruiters and carted Rebecca off to see various colleges play; and those social studies and English teachers who drew the best from Rachel. I recall Bob Lawless, the basketball coach who taught my 6′11″ son to shoot over a taller opponent by holding a broom in front of Jason's face during practice. I am grateful for the teachers who not only helped the kids develop skills but a love of learning.

Although I often urge parents to advocate for their children, it is always on the assumption that they are working hard at parenting as well. Educators frequently voice frustration about the lack of respect and common courtesy once considered routine among students. "Thank you's" are now a rare commodity. Table manners are frequently absent. Along with relaxed-fit jeans and relaxed codes of conduct have come blurred boundaries between kids and adults. I have witnessed students rummaging through a teacher's personal belongings. I have heard Beavis and Butthead-inspired comments addressed to teachers and parents. I have encountered parents who become paralyzed at the thought of reprimanding, limiting, or saying "No" to their children.

Five or six years ago I had a conversation with the mother of a thirteen-year-old boy who was acting up at home. She told me that the night before, her son had told her in no uncertain terms what she could do to herself. She was proud of the fact that she had remained calm and talked to him quietly as she watched him slam his way out of the house. I sat in disbelief. I couldn't imagine calm in my house under those circumstances. I asked her if she had gone after him. "What could I do?" she replied helplessly. I cringed, muttering to myself sarcastically, "What about tackling him on the front lawn and dragging him back into the house!" A friend of mine who is a high school counselor made an observation recently. "A number of parents today 'enable' their children to the extent that they allow them to fix the blame rather than help them fix the problem."

I always felt that our neighbors used to run and hide when they saw me coming with my soapbox, ready to pontificate on child development. Still, Dennis and I have no magic answer to child rearing. People may be taken by the young woman they read about in the papers. She is not perfect and neither are we. We cringed at some of the behavior our children brought home and we rallied our talents to combat negative influences. Sometimes what we did worked and sometimes it didn't. Despite all the books one reads, parenting is sometimes a seat-of-the-pants business. I remember an eight-year-old Rebecca running down the stairs to complain that Rachel had just called her a f—ing a———. I was *beyond* upset. She didn't learn such language from us. I summoned my elder daughter downstairs and, mustering all of my newly acquired counseling skills, I patiently explained to Rachel that we do not use such words. I didn't want to hear them ever again. "Words can be hurtful, especially to people we love," I pointed out. Rachel stood there, eyes downcast, and nodded in thoughtful agreement. Well done, I thought. Two nights later, I was standing at the bottom of the stairs, bellowing my demand that Rachel come down this instant. She had done it again. No more Mrs. Nice-Nice.

"Didn't I talk to you the other night about calling your sister bad names? Didn't I tell you I wouldn't tolerate it?" My eyes narrowed. She hung her head.

"I feel like cracking your behind. The only reason I won't swat you is because I'm afraid I won't stop. That's how angry I am. Now go to your room." Slowly she trudged upstairs. "Well," I thought to myself. "Let's see how well that works."

My deliberate use of rage worked in this instance. I wouldn't recommend this as a general practice as children will stop hearing you if anger becomes commonplace. Discipline must be crafted to fit the occasion. Sometimes less is more. One afternoon Den was home early from school because he wasn't feeling well. Hearing the school bus, Den went to the window to watch Rachel disembark. It was a tender, Kodak moment until a little boy flipped her the bird from a bus window. Stunned, Dennis watched Rachel respond in kind. He was in a dither when I arrived home. What to do! Realizing he had been an unsuspecting voyeur in a kid's world, we decided to do nothing. After all, a friend said, wasn't it better that Rachel had stood her ground and stuck up for herself rather than going to pieces? I still get a laugh recalling the look on Den's face as he recounted his afternoon shock.

It's not too different in the classroom. Sometimes you go by your gut. Just like at home, kids challenge and test, and in a split second you pull a solution out of your bag of tricks and hope that it works. Many years ago I inadvertently called a kid by his last name, having heard his classmates do it so often that it just slipped out. To my amazement he told me to shut up. I couldn't believe my ears.

"What did you say?"

"Shut up, Mrs. Lobo," he repeated.

Throw him out of the class, lecture him, or have a hissy fit? I decided to maintain decorum.

"See me after class."

Later, as we sat and talked, I discovered that problems at home were interfering with his getting along with his parents and his friends in class. I never would have learned of this if I had my hissy fit. A call home, a talk with his parents calmed his frustrations.

I love to work with parents and kids who recognize that we are in this together. It is inspiring to see the results when teachers, parents, and students strive toward common goals and achieve them. Without the cooperative efforts of parents, teachers, and the community-at-large, our children are at the mercy of greed-driven hawkers of *things*. Schools are not worlds unto themselves. Sexually explicit and violent music, computer programs, movies, and television shows desensitize our kids to the value of less lurid human qualities and often teachers see what this means firsthand.

When we, as parents, complain to producers, we hear that it is our job to monitor a child's viewing or use of the product. And what of Calvin Klein ads on billboards and city buses? Do we clap our hands over our children's eyes? I don't think we are talking about censorship. In a grown-up, responsible society, we all need to think beyond the clink of the cash register to the repercussions of our actions. A responsible television company simply refrains from airing inappropriate programming during prime time. Responsible actors and actresses who thump the drum for AIDS or drug awareness should model lifestyles that enforce their message. Responsible advertisers have to look beyond the bottom line to the effects of their advertising, the programming they support, and the products they sell. As responsible voters we should not let our politicians get away with posturing and self-serving political rhetoric.

Editorials and articles blame today's educators for lower test scores, unprepared graduates, and an unskilled workforce, but schools cannot carry the burden alone. I have seen in the eyes of children the worry that comes when businesses begin downsizing, a fancy term that translates to stress and fear when overheard by a twelve-year-old. I have heard the longing for family unity that has dissolved over the years because jobs take parents away from home for long periods of time. I have agonized over kids left unsupervised because the workplace refuses flexible hours to encourage parents to spend more time with their children. I have witnessed family members transformed into isolated units because we demand a marketplace open twenty-four hours a day, seven days a week.

And all the education in the world will not prevent teenage sexual activity or drug and alcohol use when adults display such behavior. Obscene language and violence cannot be controlled within school walls when it is out of control in our cities and neighborhoods, in our homes, and in youthful imaginations infected by commercial exploitation. Like a child in the hormonal grip of adolescence, our society is reaping the rewards of behavior left unchecked. Rebelling against authority, thumbing our nose at tradition, we are being crushed by a monster of our own making and the schools are being asked to destroy the monster. It is ludicrous to expect our schools to counteract every social ill that arises. It cannot be done. We are slapping on Band-Aids at an alarming rate, but the wound beneath does not heal. I am wearied by the onslaught of criticism aimed at dedicated and overburdened educators by politicians, disgruntled parents, the media, business, and industries. Educators do not need criticism; they need help.

For every classroom minute spent bolstering tender egos and images, there are hundreds of commercials that reduce the human being to a sex object. For every lesson on nutrition, there are countless promotions for the long and lean look that lead directly to eating disorders. For each word of praise commending intellectual prowess, there is endless worship of beauty and brawn.

I hope we can return a sense of childhood to our children. It will take more than catchy phrases or finger pointing. It will require commitment by everyone in society to put the needs of children before the almighty dollar. It will mean that those without school children join forces with parents in demanding and supporting top quality education. It will necessitate a willingness to assume responsibility for the effect we have on others whether we write songs, produce movies, sell products, parent, or teach.

As I tuck my soapbox under my arm, I challenge each of us to rethink how our lifestyles, decisions, and priorities impact children. There are no easy answers to the world's ills, but each of us can make a difference. I have already discovered that a phone call or a letter to an advertiser, company, or television station can get results. Boycotting a product that exploits children or women in its advertising is equally effective. Being brave enough to discipline ourselves and our children isn't easy in a world that has too long emphasized self-indulgence. Reclaiming a world where children once felt safe can happen if, like the UConn's women's team, we work at it one day at a time.

★ 9 ★

God's Plan

★ *REBECCA*

When I was a little girl I had the blind faith of a child. I was taught that God exists and that I should love Him, and I did. I was taught that God died for me, that He was kind and loving, and that's how I saw Him. It's how I still see Him. In my bedroom my mother hung a picture of a guardian angel protecting two young children crossing a dangerous bridge. When the going gets rough, I imagine her there, hanging over me. (Not Mom, the guardian angel.)

Like most kids I didn't enjoy Sunday School or Saturday morning catechism class. I did like our family priest, Father Menges, (who, on holy days, used to give our family an extra dousing of holy water; no doubt we needed it) and, the Sisters of St. Joseph confessed to having prayed fervently on our behalf as they watched the NCAA championship. Still, I only attended Mass because my parents didn't give me a choice of how to spend Sunday morning. I viewed my confirmation more as the end to the years of catechism than an understanding and acceptance of God. By the time I was in high school, I attended Mass more as a duty to fulfill, a habit that had been established in the first sixteen years of my life. Yet there has never been a moment when I haven't believed in Him.

One of my mother's close friends tells me each time she sees me, "God has a plan for you, Rebecca." I hope she's right. I hope I'll be able to follow His wishes. It seems as if my life so far has followed some mysterious course that I couldn't have mapped out more perfectly in my wildest fantasies in my family driveway. It hasn't been without trouble. It hasn't been without hurt and pain. I just hope and pray that I live the way I'm supposed to and follow whatever plan there is for me. For if God indeed laid those plans, I can't go wrong.

But I have gone wrong at times. When people say, "I hope my daughter grows up to be just like you," I want them to know that although I think I'm a good person, I'm not untarnished. Sometimes I wish I could go back and be a kid again. There's such an innocence and unself-consciousness in childhood. I also wish I could go back to certain parts of my life and take back things that I have done, just like everybody, I'm sure. Dig deep enough and you find everyone has things that she wishes she could change, and I'm no different. In order to move on from my mistakes, I feel the need for forgiveness from God. I never saw Him as wrathful, looking to punish me, but as eager to forgive. Because God knows exactly what I'm thinking and feeling, He knows when I'm sincerely sorry. This has always been a comfort in my life.

I wish it were as easy for people to forgive as I imagine it is for God. Everyone makes mistakes, and yet it is possible to grow beyond them, to become a great person. If you do something bad, it doesn't mean you're bad. If you're in a tough situation, you just have to work through it. If you've hurt someone, you need to do what you can to make that person feel better. But if it involves just you, you need to work it out alone. You need to remember that you are still a good person and not let your regrets overshadow that. Sometimes it's hard, the pain can stay with you for a while. But as long as you keep on working at being a good person, and you learn from your mistakes, you're moving forward.

Talking about God sometimes makes others uncomfortable. This is not my intention; God is a presence in my heart and I feel it is important to acknowledge the place He has in my life. I remember when I was a freshman or sophomore in high school, and I had to get up to say thank you's for some award. I knew that when I got to the part of thanking God I would get nervous. I wasn't comfortable speaking in front of people as it was, and I imagined they would make fun of me if I brought Him up. Of course no one ever did but I still worried. I don't anymore.

Having a faith is what saves some people from going absolutely crazy. When my mom was sick, I had complete faith in God that she was going to be okay, that she would be cured. I never cursed Him, but I did ask Him to help her fight her battle. If my mom's cancer came back, I still wouldn't blame God. But I'm totally convinced that it won't. Still, if her cancer did come back, it's something I know is out of her hands, mine, and everybody else's. You have to give the control to somebody, and I've chosen to give my faith to God. There is no stronger arm than prayer.

I prayed a lot when my mother was battling for her life, and I realized how inconsequential some of my own battles were. If things were going bad for me on the basketball court, I used to call home and talk to my parents about it. After my mom got sick, I realized how silly it must have seemed to her; I'm sure she wished her biggest problem was how things were going for me on the court. My mother became much more spiritual after her cancer. She had always been a spiritual person, but when she started going through it all, she really just gave her life to God. She doesn't let unimportant things bother her now; she doesn't get frustrated as easily and she's learned to let things roll off her. I've also learned to let the other things slide. Sometimes parents do things that embarrass their children but after the cancer my attitude was "Go ahead and embarrass me." I know now it's important to let my parents know how much I love them because the day is going to come when I will no longer be able to do that.

I always pray before I go to sleep. If I wake up and there's something troubling me, I'll pray again. If Dave and I are having an argument, I'll pray that things will resolve themselves in whatever way they're supposed to, but I won't pray for him to see things my way. If I'm having a tough day on the court, I'll pray to keep a positive outlook. I have confidence that whatever happens is for a reason and will end up being something positive in the long run. Before a game I usually pray that no one gets injured. I never ask, "Help us win this game," although I may pray for Him to help me play to the best of my ability. If we lose, I never say, "God, why did we lose?" Or I'll pray for patience when I don't feel like signing autographs. Even little things like that find me asking for help from God. In prayer I feel like I'm talking to a very patient and close friend.

And for this friend, I want nothing more than to use wisely the talents and gifts given me. Whenever people comment on my life, they marvel at how "perfectly" things fell into place. I don't chalk it up to luck and hard work as most people might. I chose the University of Connecticut over my parents' objections because I knew in my heart that it was the place for me. I remember praying to God to help me make my college decision. I felt, too, that we were destined to win the national championship. Right after the season ended I was contacted by Reebok and I needed an agent to work out the details of the shoe contract. Coach Auriemma recommended someone he knew from his days coaching at Virginia. I got in touch with this attorney and have spoken to him daily ever since. I don't believe luck placed Kenton Edelin in my path. Nor do I think I was simply in the right place at the right time with the formation of the first USA National Team.

The adage in America is that you will be rewarded for how hard you work. It is the same message that many coaches constantly feed their players. The problem is that not everyone starts in the same place. In basketball, the hardest working player on the team may sit on the bench if someone else had more height, strength, or athletic ability. In life, the hardest working kid may fall short of the tuition money needed to go to college, whereas another student, with less drive, will only have to watch his parents make a bank withdrawal. There is no ignoring the fact that some people start life with many advantages while others have none. Not everyone is rewarded for working hard and not everyone is punished for being lazy. Life would seem a little more fair if this were the case. But everyone is equal in God's eyes, and working hard with the talents He has given you is a reward in itself. It's something you can control and you always want to prepare yourself the best way you know how. That way you will have no regrets. No matter what advantages or disadvantages you had when you started out, you'll have no regrets.

There are those who doubt God exists when they see suffering in the world. I didn't see a lot of suffering when I was growing up. Southwick is a small town and is not near enough to a big city or depressed area where there is poverty. When I was about seven years old, I saw my first homeless person. I was with my brother, sister, and grandfather in Boston. I remember a man coming up and asking us for money. Even though it was mid-July, he was dressed in a long winter coat. My grandfather ignored him and told us to keep walking. As we walked away, I turned around and saw the man sit down on a piece of cardboard against a brick building. My grandfather explained that the man was homeless and the reason he did not give him any money was that he would just use it to buy liquor. Obviously, I was too young to understand why this man was living on the street. In my young mind, he became a bum.

After four years of college and many sociology and political science courses, I have a better understanding of why this man was begging for money on the street. God is not responsible for this man's suffering, we all are. I hope I never take for granted the privileges my parents provided. I also hope that I will always feel a chill and my head will tell me something is not right when I see a person on the street who must beg for money to survive. No one should have to live like this in the wealthiest country in the world. No one should be forced to have their biggest goal in life be mere survival.

When I was little, the solution seemed obvious. I thought it made sense to tax most those people who had a lot of money. I didn't quite understand how rich people could be so selfish and fight so hard against giving the government money. It just seemed logical to take money from the rich and give it to the poor. Ever since I started getting paychecks, my feelings have changed a bit. Things are not as black and white to me as they were when I was a kid. I guess I understand how the system works. I may not like it, but I understand it. Maybe someday, with God's help, I can help change it.

★ *RUTHANN*

During my childhood, the center of Medfield was marked by four church steeples that rose heavenward within a few short blocks of each other. They could have been fortifications so separate were they from one another. Unlike the camaraderie that exists among many faiths today, the clergy and members of the various churches in Medfield never, to my recollection, came together on a spiritual level (and they were all Christians!). Although I attended Sunday Mass at St. Edward's Church with my mother, my formal religious training was restricted to classes for first communion and confirmation. Nevertheless, I prayed nightly and never doubted that my words were heard. I treasured those rare times when I found myself in a nearly empty church where I could contemplate God and my relationship with Him.

Sundays were always earmarked for worship and family relaxation. After church, we enjoyed a breakfast of bacon and eggs, toast, juice, and coffee, prepared with expert results by my dad. The Sunday papers were divided among family members according to interests. Later, the family sat down to Sunday dinner, a feast of Mom's creation complete with a roast, gravy, mashed potatoes, salad, rolls, vegetables, and dessert. The remainder of the day was devoted to board games, reading, outdoor activities, or an afternoon movie. My overriding memory is one of serenity and quiet. There was no rushing around to malls (they didn't exist) or sports practices (there were none). There were no meals caught on the run. It was understood that Sunday was a day for God and family.

In my mind's eye, God took the shape of an all-powerful being "out there somewhere." He loomed larger than life when I did something wrong, and I became anxious when I contemplated His knowing everything I did. I could not imagine God's loving me enough to intervene in my life unless I was very good and I prayed a whole lot! My view softened in the quiet of my room as I knelt by my bed at night and offered up my prayers.

In marriage, Den and I shared our beliefs and passed on the traditions of our Christian faith to our children. We both taught religious education; I sang in the choir and Den became a lector. We began taking Jason to church when he was old enough to sit quietly during Mass. Each Sunday we told him, "We are going to pray to God."

One morning after Mass, as we stood outside the church, Jason noted some parishioners in conversation with our priest. He asked, "Why are all those people talking to God?" Better set that one straight!

Our Marriage Encounter in 1976 not only cemented our relationship with each other, it added a new dimension to my relationship with God. As the weekend drew to a close, I wrote to Dennis:

My Dear Husband,

Since this weekend, God seems more real to me. I feel like someone who has repeatedly been told something but didn't fully believe it until she saw it herself. I feel like someone who has been told how good a certain dish will taste; I imagined its flavor but didn't truly know until I ate it myself. I feel as if we are a part of God's plan.

God has been good to us in so many ways. He has guided us and helped us learn by trial and error as all good parents help their children learn. In return, I feel gratitude and the willingness to love Him completely as I love you. If He can love us as we love one another, then we can't do less in return.

I feel peaceful when I think of God as a member of our family. I feel safe in the knowledge that He is there always. I feel a willing obligation to do His will so that we may be in His grace and love forever.

Lovingly yours,
Me

After that weekend it was as if God had moved from the Heavens and now stood in our midst with His arms around the two of us. For ten years following our Marriage Encounter weekend, Den and I met once a month with other couples who had joined us on that weekend. We shared the intimacies of our lives and forged a bond that surpasses time and distance.

Surprisingly, I later experienced a similar spiritual bonding through basketball. During our second trip to the AAU (Amateur Athletic Union) National Championship games in Charleston, West Virginia, two other mothers and I agreed to meet before each game and pray for good sportsmanship and protection from injury on both sides. Before the week was out, we were eight or nine women in number. We read and discussed scripture, prayed together, and established a pattern for subsequent tournaments.

As I grew older, I no longer looked to the heavens to find Him; I looked in my heart. Like any relationship, mine with God needed tending in order to develop and flourish. Although my belief in God remained constant, my willingness to nurture my faith faded in and out depending on the demands of my life at the moment. Too often, I allowed the hustle and bustle of being a wife, parent, and teacher to overshadow my relationship with my faith and my God. I was caught up in the daily hubbub of my job, household chores, political commitments, and basketball rigors. Routine challenges took on the enormity of major crises: clashing points of view at work, my daughter Rachel's decision to change colleges, unexpected company, requests for basketball tickets. The days blended into each other as I scurried from one task to another. Busy, busy, busy. My self-appointed task was to keep it all in order; to stay in control. Although I knew Jesus was still in my heart, He had to share space with an increasing number of worries, concerns, projects, and desires. The demands of the world became so loud that I couldn't always hear my Savior's voice. I never doubted He was there for me, but I took Him for granted.

And then the cancer came.

In the snap of a finger I faced my own mortality eye to eye. I had to ask myself some difficult questions. Had I spent enough time with my children? Had I taught them the lessons they needed to know? Had I told my parents and brother how much I loved them? Had I taken every opportunity to laugh with, make love with my husband? Had I led a life pleasing to my God?

It's funny how quickly a crisis can draw a person up short and force her to separate the wheat from the chaff. It's as if I put my entire life in a giant sieve, gave it a few vigorous shakes, and discovered a very small number of priorities remaining. I had to face the hard truth that I had wasted time and energy on many things that really didn't matter. While my husband slept beside me, I wept in my solitude for opportunities never taken with friends and loved ones.

Although surrounded by people who loved me, I felt desperately alone at the time. The demons of fear fought for my soul. As ludicrous as it sounds today, I wasn't sure if I could live with the terrible fear I had of dying. Initially, I was powerless and out of control. I needed to come to grips with this disease called cancer. The medical profession offered its best treatment. I was grateful. But what I needed most was hope. Turning to my Bible, I grasped for solace. I flipped through the pages, and as if written in boldfaced type, the words of Isaiah 41:10 leapt out at me. "Do not be afraid, for I am with you; stop being anxious and watchful, for I am your God. I give you strength, I bring you help, I uphold you with my victorious right hand." I armed myself with this particular piece of scripture. I read it in the morning. I read it on the way to basketball games. I read it while traveling to the doctor's office. I read it through the tears of my despair. The passage continued: "Fear not, for I am with you: I am your God."

My friend Kathy arrived at my house shortly after my surgery. She presented me with a set of tapes on healing. The primary message was to focus not on the disease but on God. Not always an easy task. My mind wandered endlessly to the state of my health and each time I battled the resurgence of fear. Somewhere in those tapes a message appeared that was restated in the books and other tapes I began to devour: II Timothy 1:7, "For God hath not given us the spirit of fear but of power, and love, and of a sound mind."

I looked for God and He was there. Initially, I clung to Him in desperation. I fretted and wailed and begged God to heal me. In Psalm 46:10, He told me, "Be still and know that I am God." I listened and quieted. I sought His counsel wherever I could find it. I found Him in the faces of my family, colleagues, friends, and students. I found Him in the notes from strangers. I found Him in the Sunday Mass in my home parish, Our Lady of the Lake, and I found Him in the healing services of many denominations. I found Him in my weekly prayer meetings with Pat Joy, the deacon of Trinity Episcopal Church in Tariffville, Connecticut. I came to realize that throughout the years when there had been distance between God and me, it wasn't God who had moved.

I no longer seek God simply for the healing of my body, I seek God for the healing of my soul. I realize that my focus has shifted from the disease to God, and with that shift comes great joy and peace. I can state with conviction that my Lord has carried me through this ordeal. Now I am more responsible in the care of my relationship with God. In addition to weekly worship, I have tried to include daily readings and prayer. I attend a women's group devoted to spiritual development every Monday night. An unlikely group of varying ages and educational and economic backgrounds, we bring our struggles and triumphs along with our eccentricities as we strive to know Him better. Along with prayer and scripture, we have debated topics as far afield as the trumped up merits of the Wonder Bra. The ring of our frequent laughter, including the night one woman inadvertently wore another's coat home (car keys in pocket), reminds me that God has a sense of humor!

I liken my relationship with God to being able to see the three-dimensional picture in the Magic-Eye pictures created by the computer. For over a year I had stared at those pictures only seeing one-dimensional views. When my kids asked if I could see the picture, I honestly answered yes. I thought I saw what I was supposed to be seeing. It was only after mastering the technique of viewing the pictures, however, that I realized what I had been missing. The picture had been there all the time, but I just hadn't seen it. So it was with God. He has always been there. I thought I could see Him; then suddenly, I saw Him in a new dimension. He gives me love, He gives me power, He gives me hope.

I am grateful for the weakening of those fortifications that prevented me from entering the other churches in Medfield while I was growing up. The bonds we share in faith are far greater than our differences. When God reached out to me through others, I did not stop to ask their church affiliation. I thankfully accepted their prayers as well as their kindnesses and love.

During the past two years, I have often wondered how anyone can endure a crisis without faith. I think young people in particular have a great hunger for spiritual fulfillment. When that hunger is not met by one of the world's great religions, it is often met by the gods of addiction, materialism, or cult worship. This was never made clearer to me than at a conference for professional counselors who work with young women; it was sponsored by a nationally renowned and respected organization. As the morning speaker, a psychotherapist, gave her presentation, she revealed that she was a witch, albeit a "good witch." I cringed. Some participants were agitated; others hung on her every word. Those with a void in their lives were openly willing to fill it by embracing her views. "At what cost?" I thought. "And with whom will they share these views?"

I have also noted a reluctance by the media to include any reference to the presence of God in Rebecca's or my life. During my countless interviews, I never failed to mention the spiritual support at the core of my family. I never forgot to tell them that in crisis my strength came from God. Rarely did those comments appear in print or on the evening news.

More important than tossing a ball through a hoop or earning a place on the school honor roll is a spiritual foundation from which to draw strength and moral fortitude. Imbedded in such a foundation is the well from which we drink when we are stripped naked and faced with our nothingness. My wish is for families to reclaim their responsibility to provide and nurture the spiritual development of their children in the house of worship of their choice. It is a deeper well than one might ever imagine.

★ 10 ★

An Uncle Wiggley Adventure

★ *REBECCA*

Homecoming. The much anticipated return of Rebecca Lobo to Gampel Pavilion at the University of Connecticut.

Anticipated by me, of course. The weekend of November 5, 1995 was a date that had been circled on my calendar since the day I left Storrs for the Olympic training center in Colorado Springs. This was the day that the USA Basketball National Team, the core of the team that would go to the Atlanta Olympics in the summer of 1996, would play the UConn Huskies. The trip to Storrs was part of our cross-country tour of exhibition games against the finest women's college basketball teams in the country, a season intended to make the USA National Team a real team, not just a group of professional basketball stars thrown together three months before the Olympics. But in Colorado Springs and on the road, I wasn't always thinking about Atlanta. I was thinking about November 5, the Sunday I was to return home to play my former teammates in front of all the Connecticut faithful in Gampel. As the date approached, it felt like years had passed since I had last played there. In reality, I had left Storrs barely five weeks before.

When the time had finally come to leave Storrs for Colorado, I was beside myself. I was flying to a state very far away, I was leaving my best friends and teammates, my family was no longer right next door, and for the first time in my life I had to say good-bye to a boyfriend. Dave and I enjoyed a great summer, spending every spare minute we had together. Whatever we were doing, even if it was just watching television or walking around campus, I had been content and happy.

Of course, that had made the idea of leaving home so much more difficult to contemplate. Whenever reference was made to September 26, I couldn't help but feel glum. The week before I left was extremely difficult. I wanted to savor every second, but a million demands were placed on my time. One day I was in Los Angeles filming a Reebok commercial, two days later I was in New York City for a photo shoot, the next day I was in southern Connecticut doing a commercial for the regional Chevrolet dealers. Eight hours later I was headed to Boston for an all-day appearance. And when, finally, I returned home, I was extremely tired. I wanted to spend time with Dave but just ended up falling asleep as we watched television. Finally, that Friday I went home because my mother and I had an interview. As I walked through the door I broke down. Exhausted and frustrated, I felt like I had no time for myself or anyone close to me. As before, I felt like a puppet going wherever I was pulled.

Mom and Dad listened to me and gave me the thing I needed most, a hug. My mom also wanted to call my agent and give him a piece of her mind for doing this to me right before I left. But it was not Kenton's fault. I had obligations to fill, and the timing was just awful. My frame of mind was abysmal. Besides that, my basketball suffered; I didn't have as much time to work out, and when I got a spare second, all my body could do was sleep. This sort of life just leaves me feeling worn down and miserable. I've sworn it will never happen again.

Plus, I still had to deal with leaving Storrs and leaving all my friends. I met Coach Dailey for brunch and went to Coach Auriemma's house to say good-bye. I had sought the opinions, approval, and advice of these two people so often that it was hard to imagine not seeing them everyday. My parents came with me to Dave's first football game of the season that last weekend (UConn won on his game-winning kick with only six seconds left) and they got to meet his parents for the first time. It was a great night. The next night I went out to dinner with Jen Rizzotti. We had eaten almost every meal together for the last three years, seen each other every day, talked about *everything*. We went to Friendly's and sat and talked. When I dropped her off at her dorm, I lost it. Jen is very emotional so we tried to say good-bye as quickly as possible. We didn't want to be slobbering fools because neither of us had thought to bring tissues. Just when I had regained my composure, I read the card she gave me and broke down again. The next day I had to say good-bye to Dave. When he hugged me, I didn't want him to let go. When I saw tears in his eyes, I realized I was not the only one having a hard time. That's when it dawned on me that sometimes you have to say good-bye. It didn't matter that both of us wanted to stay together, in the same place at the same time. There was something bigger each of us had to do. We couldn't spend all of our time together anymore. Our feelings for each other wouldn't lessen, but we had to say good-bye. No matter how much it hurt, it had to be done.

I was so absorbed with saying good-bye to my friends at school that I didn't leave much time to say good-bye to my family. When you leave a place you've been for a while, there's always the fear that things will be different when you return. The one constant for me is and always has been my family. Because they have always been there, I sometimes worry that I take their presence for granted. Mom drove me to the airport and Dad met us there. When I got to the ticket counter, someone working for another airline came over and gave me a note from my coaches. It said, "Smile. You'll always be a Husky." I still carry that note in my jacket pocket. At the gate I was a sobbing fool. A man came over and asked for my autograph, but the minute he saw my face, I know he regretted it.

Walking down the runway onto the plane was like walking from one life to the next, and I was scared. I was going to a new life I knew nothing about. I had no idea what to expect in Colorado. I didn't know what to expect from basketball, my teammates, coaches, or anything else. I was twenty-one years old, and I was finally leaving home.

* * * *

The difference between men's and women's basketball is not in the level of excitement. The technical differences are only in the size of the ball (ours is a little smaller) and the amount of time on the shot clock (we have thirty seconds to get a shot off each offensive possession whereas the men have thirty-five). If people want to see numerous dunks or high flying acrobatics then they might be disappointed with the women's game. However, if they want to see five people playing together, relying on each other to get open and stop the other team, then they will appreciate our game. If they want to see people fundamentally sound in the game of basketball—setting screens and playing team defense—then they will appreciate our game. If they want to see people willing to give all of themselves, shedding blood, sweat, and tears every time they step on the court, they will appreciate our game. And if they want to see people playing basketball for pure joy and not the possibility of a pot of gold at the end of the rainbow, then they will *love* our game.

During my four years in college, women's basketball saw media interest and fan enthusiasm erupt. The first time I saw UConn play in 1990, they didn't even have all the bleachers pulled out. There were about two thousand fans in the stands. In contrast, my senior year we sold out almost every home game (that's almost nine thousand people) and even had people scalping tickets. Our championship game against Tennessee had higher television ratings in Connecticut than the Super Bowl. If I had played ten or even five years earlier, the same player on the same team, with the exact same record, my story would be very different. Maybe I would have been on a team that won the national championship, but the game wouldn't have been seen by very many people. There would have been no sneaker contract, no invitation to appear on *The Late Show with David Letterman*, and I'm dead certain I wouldn't be writing this book.

Training with me in Colorado were the women who had blazed that trail. I couldn't help but be intimidated by the prospect of playing with them. I went from being one of the oldest members and cocaptain of a college team to being the rookie among the best women basketball players in the world. I was no longer playing with college students who had yet to own a car or live in an apartment. Because the United States doesn't have a professional women's basketball league, my new teammates had had to leave the country and play overseas. They were women who had been all around the world, who had played for many different coaches. In less than a year, I had gone from listening to seventeen-year-old teammates talk about leaving their high school sweethearts to hearing women plan their weddings. Purchasing a minirefrigerator or a cordless telephone was not quite as big a deal with the USA team as it had been for us at UConn. Their concerns ranged from paying the mortgage to selecting furniture for the house. Katrina McClain and Theresa Edwards were both over thirty and Sheryl Swoopes and Ruthie Bolton-Holyfield were already married. Sheryl's husband of three months actually moved out to Colorado Springs to be with her.

I was the first to arrive. When I got to Colorado Springs, I was picked up from the airport and driven to my new "home." Reebok had provided a very nice apartment for Jennifer Azzi and me. It had two bedrooms and two bathrooms, and was fully furnished. Towels were neatly laid out on the racks and fresh sheets were on the bed. We even had cable and, thank God, I thought as I dialed Dave, the phone worked. I was extremely excited to see a washer and dryer hidden behind two doors. Imagine my surprise when I realized that, unlike college, you didn't have to pay to use them. Just like home.

I walked across the street to McDonald's to get something to eat. When I returned, the apartment was still empty. I spent the better part of the day on the phone with Rachel and Dave. I really didn't know what to do with myself; I was lost. The closest basketball hoop was a fifteen minute drive away and I had left my car in Connecticut. Finally, Jennifer and the rest of the team arrived. Everyone had an apartment in the same complex. Most of our teammates lived on our floor. It was almost like being back in the dorm with my UConn teammates. Almost.

I was very lucky to have Jennifer as a roommate. For the first few weeks, she really looked out for me. For four years at Stanford, she had played for Tara Vanderveer, the woman who coaches the Olympic team, and she had played overseas. The coaches didn't arrive until that weekend, so the players had a chance to get together beforehand and play pickup. We then had orientation: a day of media training; a meeting going over rules and regulations about behavior, dress, and travel; and a trip to Denver and the Nicole Miller boutique so we could get outfitted for gowns for the Women's Sports Foundation dinner that we were all to attend in New York City three weeks later.

When we had free time, I usually just went back to the apartment. I was a bit homesick, but being busy and around my teammates made life a lot easier. One night the team went to the movies, but I stayed in to collect my thoughts. It was awkward for me because everyone else on the team had played together in previous summers, and they knew each other well. They didn't know me. They were all very nice, and friendly too, but I guess developing a relationship just takes time. Even when the team hung out in someone's room, I generally stayed in the apartment and talked on the phone or worked on my writing. I didn't yet feel like I could be my smart-ass self around my new teammates. So I kept to myself. I wasn't trying to be antisocial. I just felt out of place. I was still hanging on to the life I had back home.

The first day of practice is always difficult. No one on the team really knows what to expect from the coaches or anyone else. We practiced for three hours and I proved why I was given the nickname "rookie." I messed up some drills, did okay in others. The high altitude in Colorado made it difficult for everyone on the team to catch her breath. The fact that I missed some workouts over the summer because of travel and appearances made it even more difficult. Three times a week, we had an hour of weight lifting. The morning after our first timed run on the track, I found myself along with six teammates doing extra conditioning at 8 A.M. It turned out that over the summer we had all filled out our workout sheets incorrectly. For each error, there was an hour of work to be made up.

It takes a long time for a coach to take the full measure of a player and for a player to take the full measure of a coach. I didn't expect to have the same relationship with Coach Vanderveer as I had with Coach Auriemma. Yet, I couldn't stop myself from noticing the differences in style, philosophy, and manner. At the same time, I couldn't help but be reminded of my first year at UConn, trying to rid myself of that "freshman feeling," and trying to understand why Coach was coming down so hard on me. Once again I told myself, I was the player and she was the coach, off court and on.

* * * *

Thirty-nine days later I was back in Storrs. I really didn't know what it would feel like to play against Jen Rizzotti and Jamelle Elliott instead of with them. It was the one game on the tour I most longed to play, but it was also the game I didn't want to play. I sensed that things were going to be different almost immediately. As I got off of Route 84 on Saturday night, I saw the sign that said "University of Connecticut Home of the 1995 Women's Basketball National Champions" that had been put up the day we returned from Minneapolis. Five miles later there hung another, newly made, sign: "Rebecca and the national team: beware of the dog." One sign reminded me of a wonderful past, the other made me feel completely weird. I felt odd, like a stranger. Perhaps that was a good thing.

I was also anticipating my reunion with Dave. That first night back we had only forty-five minutes together. It seemed like I had only been there a minute when it was time to leave and meet my team. As luck would have it, I was five minutes late and had to pay a $10 fine to USA basketball. The next day I was able to see Dave for a grand total of twenty minutes. His team was staying at a hotel about twenty miles away because they had a game the next day and the coach wanted to take them away from the "distractions of campus life." I arrived at his hotel at 10:30 P.M. after his meetings were over and left before his eleven o'clock curfew. We had to meet in the lobby because the team was not allowed to have "girls" in their rooms. We went around the corner and sat down on a window sill hoping that we'd have some privacy and a chance to talk. Three times people came up to us asking for my autograph. (I still wonder how it could be possible that there is a single soul in Connecticut without my signature.) I have to give Dave credit for putting up with all this. Perhaps, too, I should have been thankful for these interruptions. We had both been feeling the strain of separation.

The next day Dave had a home game on the UConn campus, but I didn't have even ten minutes to watch. I started off the morning at 8 A.M. with a Reebok clinic and was then driven to Hartford for a USA basketball clinic and autograph signing.

Following the signing I had just enough time to grab a quick lunch before signing more autographs at a local department store. Then a press conference was immediately followed by practice and another autograph session before hitting the weight room. After finding out the final score of Dave's game (they won), I rushed back to campus where my former teammates were getting together to have a ceremonial dinner. We were to be presented with our national championship rings.

I walked through the door at 7:30 P.M. I knew where I stood when the first thing I heard was Jamelle holler out, "We're gonna kick your butt tomorrow, Rebecca!" I just smiled and gave everyone hugs. They made a few inside jokes that I didn't get. They talked about what happened at practice that day and other days. I didn't love my ex-teammates any less, it was just *different*. We were going through different things. After the dinner we were presented with our championship rings. They were gold and had a blue stone. On top of the stone was a number one with five diamonds in it. On the sides of the ring it said 35-0, perfect, teamwork, Big East champs, and my number (50). They were really beautiful. What they signified was even better than a perfect record. The memories, and (if I'm not a klutz) my ring, will last forever. The season was over.

After the ring ceremony, I went to Dave's room and spent a few hours with him. We patched things up and were able to relax a little more. It was the most time we spent together the whole weekend. I had been kept so busy with appearances that I didn't even get a chance to see my parents until Sunday morning. Not quite how I had envisioned my return.

Finally Sunday, the day of the great game, arrived. It was really bizarre to walk into a different locker room and to warm up at a different basket than I was accustomed. It was even stranger to see my former team run out with the band playing the fight song. I had always gotten chills and a rush of adrenaline when I ran out to that song. Now, I just watched as they made their way onto the court. The championship banner was unfurled and I stood with the UConn team for the last time. When I was introduced, the Connecticut fans stood and cheered, giving me a great welcome. As I wasn't in a starting position, I watched the opening shots from the bench, and found myself wanting to cheer when UConn made a basket. I felt a sense of pride when they scored, but I also knew that I would try to stop them when I got in the game. (I also didn't want to run sprints next practice if we played poorly. I mean, no one said loyalty should involve sprints.) When I finally got in the game and scored, the building was silent. A year before they had applauded wildly. At one point in the second half, Kara blocked my shot and the place erupted with cheers.

It was obvious who played for UConn now, and it was obvious who didn't. If I had been playing for Connecticut and Coach Auriemma, the press wouldn't have made such a big deal about the fact that I only played a total of thirteen minutes. But because I was playing for the National Team, it made the evening news. I was disappointed by my lack of playing time, as anyone would be. I had a lot of family and friends there and wanted as much opportunity as I could get to play in front of them. But it was not to be. I never even got to say hello to my "little sister" Lauren and her little sister, Shannon, sitting in the same place under the hoop.

To be honest, I'm glad I won't play against UConn again. I want my memories from Gampel Pavilion to be of me wearing the Husky uniform. I want them to be with Coach Auriemma as my coach and the fans cheering for me instead of against me. It was great to come back "home," but on November 5, 1995, I was a visitor. My family was there but I didn't get to spend much time with them. My boyfriend was there but he had to cheer against his classmates and friends in order to root for me. My coaches and my teammates were there, but half were sitting on the opposite bench.

After the game, a reporter asked me if I had changed. Some might think that having money changes people. But to be honest, I gave all my money to a financial planner so I don't see it anyway. When we get our meal allowances on the road, I save as much as I can. I buy generic shampoo (actually, my mom still gets it for me) and love a sale at the mall as much as the next person. I guess old habits just die hard. I told the reporter the only difference between the year before and that day was that I now owned a car. I guess that wasn't completely true.

During the years I spent at UConn, I never noticed the changes I was undergoing. Being away altered that. While I was practicing that final weekend in Gampel, I knew that I no longer belonged there under the lights playing my heart out or there alone letting my mind wander. It wasn't a bad feeling at all, just a realization. When I returned to UConn, I saw the life I knew so well going on around me. People were hustling to class and mingling about. I missed it a little bit but not too much. I was glad that I wasn't studying for exams or getting up early to go to class. I enjoyed the academic part of my life there but it was nice not to be studying for the first time in sixteen years. I was glad that I could now choose the books I wanted to read.

When I was done with media interviews and my shower, I had fifteen minutes to give my family hugs before it was time to drive to the airport. As the car pulled away from the campus, it was my time to pull away too. I was finally ready to go. It was time for me to leave the past behind once and for all and arrive at the next stop on my destination. This whirlwind tour I call my life was pushing forward. I couldn't stop it, I couldn't even slow it down.

I had finally stopped trying.

* * * *

Basketball was always my escape hatch. It isn't any more. Recently, I found that I really didn't have anything to escape from in my new life. I don't have exams to stress out over, and I spend so much time working out, I don't have the time to come up with other problems. Strictly speaking, of course, that's not entirely true. I no longer have to worry about a coach getting angry if I'm late for practice, but I do have to worry about getting fined. What name brand appears on my warm-up suit is now of the essence. Since a certain apparel company is a major sponsor of the National Team, we must wear its clothes whenever we are seen in public as a team. Failure to comply results in a twenty-five dollar fine. I just hope and pray that basketball never becomes the thing I want to escape *from.* If that day ever comes, it will be the time for me to give up playing as a professional.

Although basketball is less and less of a game to me now, I still try to keep a tight hold on my priorities. God still does and always will come first. My family follows and then my friends. It's not always easy to keep that sense of balance, although I do try. I feel I'm only just beginning to understand the struggles of a working woman. I'm profoundly thankful that I was chosen to play for the National Team, and I hope that by this time next year there will be a professional women's basketball league in the United States. However, becoming a professional player takes some getting used to. I don't want to see basketball lose its true meaning for women in a rush of endorsement contracts (although the contracts are long overdue). I don't want to see women's basketball lose its meaning for those fans who were there before the sneaker companies were. It's up to the players to keep the innocence we have in our game. We're finally getting opportunities that were only available to men in the past. We must now try to ensure greater opportunities for the future. We must be responsible.

It's a pretty strange thing when the past meets the present and discusses the future! One stop on the National Team's tour was George Washington University in Washington, D.C. Along with the game came a meeting with women senators, representatives, and Supreme Court justices. I stood and mingled at a luncheon on Capitol Hill and listened to Patsy Mink, the congresswoman from Hawaii and coauthor of Title IX, talk about the constant battle she is fighting to keep it in place. I listened to Justices Sandra Day O'Connor and Ruth Bader Ginsberg talk about the exciting prospect of having more female representation on the highest court in the land. I listened in amazement as Senator Carole Moseley-Braun talked about playing basketball back in the days when women couldn't cross half-court.

I felt I was in the presence of the most powerful women in the United States. As a result of their work, especially Title IX, I had opportunities on the basketball court my mother was denied. Because of some of their work, I have a future with more open doors and fewer restrictions than my mother and grandmothers faced. As a result of their and many other women's convictions, I am able to climb the ladder of success and get closer to the glass ceiling. And as I get closer, this ceiling will be easier for me to shatter and break.

These women are doing their part in politics to make a difference, to make this country and our world a better place. Hopefully, I am doing my part, at least in the athletic realm. After all, don't women deserve it? I know my grandmothers and my mom did. I know my sister does and Lauren and Shannon. I will try to do my part. When it gets hard, I must remember the past and think of the future. One day, hopefully, my daughter will thank me. I can't help but see Lauren's painted face when I look in the mirror and put on those earrings she gave me. I don't want to let her down.

I have a deep love for this game. It has always meant so much to me, and I'm sure I will never live far from a basketball hoop. But it is not who I am. However much time and energy I put into it, basketball or any other occupation cannot define the person I am—it's just one part of me. It's a part of something much greater, but only a part nonetheless. Hopefully, young kids will think of themselves as individuals first and athletes second. Basketball could end for me tomorrow but I will continue to be Rebecca Lobo. I will continue to have the same priorities and live my life the best way I know how. I will continue to judge myself based on the person I am.

Our sport has gotten to the point where we can stand on our own. Two women's teams playing against each other can be very exciting and worth the price of admission. I am excited about the possibility of a professional league in the United States. I think the country is ready for it. I know I am. For years they have had professional ball overseas; it's a shame we don't have a league here in the country where the game was invented. I want to continue playing basketball, but I want more than anything to stay in the United States. I've never considered myself that much of a homebody. But recently I've realized how much I love being close to home.

Still, if a women's league is not successful in this country, I probably will play overseas. After my basketball career, I plan to pursue a career in sports broadcasting, doing color commentary for basketball games, especially women's. If that doesn't work out, I'm sure something else will come up. I leave it in God's hands to decide what will happen in my life. I know that as long as I do that, I cannot go wrong.

I am less afraid of change now, but I hope I never become a stranger to myself. I will grow over the years, and my life will be different with the passing of each day. I have more days ahead of me than I have behind me (which I realized every time I tried to think of material for this book). The time will come for me to pass on the lessons I have learned to a daughter or son of my own. This knowledge has nothing to do with correct shooting form or how to make a layup. It has to do with becoming the best person you can. A loving and caring individual who respects others as much as she respects herself. My mother taught me how to be that person, and I won't let her down. One day it will be my turn to try to pass that on to my child. I look forward to that day.

★ *RUTHANN*

When I was growing up, our cellarway overflowed with boxes and bags stuffed with fabric, lace, buttons, and trinkets. My mother collected and saved a variety of odds and ends, which she turned into an assortment of crafts. She stored other odds and ends, mementos of her youth, in a large cedar chest at the foot of her bed, and on occasion she unlocked the chest to reveal its treasures: faded pictures, locks of hair, a yellowed wedding dress. There was something magic in the pungent aroma of the cedar wood that filled my nostrils, and I snuggled close to catch a glimpse of the "girl" my mother had been.

Riches! Trinkets whose value rested not in the marketplace but in shared memories: a locket, a lace hankie, an unfinished quilt. "Don't sit on the bedspread, Rachel, Grandma made it! Be careful, Rebecca, that's the tea set Granny had when she was a little girl." Family histories in the making. Older traditions interwoven with new ones, new ideas, new challenges. Holiday celebrations where cookies and pretzels decorated the Christmas tree, when Santa's gifts were left unwrapped, where a piece of coal in the toe of each stocking was a reminder that there is room for personal improvement. Playground jingles sung with a naughty flair. Sauerkraut served over mashed potatoes with kielbasa (which, incidentally, induced my labor with two of my three children). Grandma . . . Mom . . . Me.

I am a sentimental woman and my mind journeys frequently over the past. Yet, through the helter-skelter of life, the Lord has a habit of bestowing little gifts that remind me to savor the present. On a cold day in November, Den and I had hurried home from school with the intention of working out at our health club. An unexpected phone call delayed us, and I lamented that the hour was too late to head out for exercise.

"Come on," Den prodded. "Put on your Reebok warm-ups and we'll go for a walk."

"Yeah, right," I answered, "and get run over in the process." It was the last day of November and the sun had long since disappeared.

"Oh, come on," he persisted, "you've got those neat little reflectors on your shoes. We'll be fine."

Grumbling all the while, I pulled on my workout clothes. "Hmm, at least I look fit," I thought as I checked my reflection in the mirror. I made sure my outfit was "light, bright, and visible at night!" Insisting that Den grab a flashlight, I prepared myself unwillingly for a half hour walk in the frozen dark. Yet, as I stepped out of the house, I discovered the glow of a nearly full moon reflecting on the first fallen snow of the season. The air was crisp but pleasing, and I tugged my woolen hat over my ears. Inwardly I delighted in the hush of the evening and the shadows of the woodland cast by moonlight. As Den and I chugged along the street, I retreated into my thoughts. "This is one of the good times," I said to myself. I glanced at my husband. "I love this man, dear Lord. Thank you for putting him in my life."

"Maybe we'll see the deer kids." Den smiled.

"Great," I answered with little enthusiasm. Conjuring up the other wildlife spotted over the years I mused, "Maybe we'll see a bear or a mountain lion." I quickened my pace.

Yet in the silence that punctuated our teasing, I savored the pleasure of the moment. "I need to enjoy each day I'm given," I reminded myself. Not an unfamiliar refrain from someone who has encountered breast cancer.

I am entering a new phase of my life. "What will you do now that the kids are grown?" "What will you do now that basketball has ended?" Familiar questions. I puzzle over my answers. I am in a constant tug-of-war recognizing that my children are grown but still wanting to protect them from the world. It is the challenge of letting go of the past and savoring the present. It is the challenge of allowing family ties to be tested and trust that the threads we have woven will hold. I have been here before.

When Jason was four weeks old, he was presented a brown teddy bear. Dubbed "Bear," this cuddly stuffed creature was soon joined by "Blanket," a soft, ecru, flannel sheet, to provide comfort to Jason at bedtime or in moments of unhappiness. Over the years, Blanket was reduced to a fistful of knotted shreds and, like the Velveteen Rabbit, Bear bore the worn spots and mended ears of a much-loved friend that somehow had been real. The day Bear was permanently moved from the bed to a shelf stirred feelings of sadness in both Den and myself. Our little boy was growing up.

The day after we had deposited Jason at Dartmouth, I returned home from work and immediately headed for the second floor and Jason's room at the top of the stairs. My gaze fell upon Bear and, sweeping him up into my arms, I listened to my own sobs break the silence. The first of my chicks had flown and it wrenched my heart.

Mentally I shook my own shoulders. "Get a grip," I scolded. "He's going off to college. It's not like he's in jail or the hospital. You should be happy." But I could also hear myself calculating the distance between Hanover, New Hampshire, and Southwick.

Watching my children leave for the world of higher education never became easier. I choked back tears each time we said our good-byes. Rachel followed Jason and set off to establish herself in college. Having been the most resistant to my prodding about her schoolwork, I was anxious about her ability to discipline herself. One night the phone rang.

"Mom, this is Rachel. I guess you know that; not too many people call you 'Mom.' (Heh heh). I have a question about a paper I'm writing."

My heart sank. "Up to her old tricks," I thought. "Doing her work at the last minute." Expecting the worst, I asked, "When is your paper due?"

"Next week."

"Next week? I expected you to say it was due tomorrow."

"This is college, Mom," she chided. "You can't leave things to the last minute in college."

So this child, too, was becoming her own person. And guess what? She was doing it without me.

Rebecca's leaving home for college was made easier knowing that she was within an hour's drive. We were not only able to see her play basketball, we were able to meet for dinner or a quick visit. Nevertheless, the quietness of the house and dinners for two left no doubt that our children were grown. In the circle of life, we had reached another turning.

Sending each child off to college marked the biggest shift in our role as parents. The bursar's office reduced our job to paying the bills; every other aspect of college life remained in the hands of the children. I find it amusing how formidably the colleges guard the privacy of our kids. Grades are sent under cover to the student, but tuition and fees are sent in duplicate to the parents. We always get stuck with the best part! Of course we were permitted to haul furnishings, suitcases, bags of groceries, and an assortment of stuffed animals back and forth over the years, but I never became completely comfortable with dormitory bulletin boards advertising free condoms and clinics on preventing date rape. What kind of world were we putting our children into? What ever happened to that safe yesteryear when a college student could get expelled for breaking curfew?

The kids stood conspicuously in front of the graffiti scribbled on the elevator walls, hiding words that might elicit from me a litany of dos and don'ts. Had Den and I armed them with enough information and good sense to stave off the evils I suddenly imagined lurking around every corner? Perhaps a lesson or two could still be taught as we walked back to the car. My kids rolled their eyes at each other in that silent, all-knowing gesture of exasperation, "Oh, Mom. Give it a rest."

The need for trips to dormitories has passed. It is a time to both reclaim and redefine myself. It is time to renew interests put on hold while caught up and carried along by the whirlwind of basketball and breast cancer. It is a time to finish knitting the sweater I started for Jason when he was still in college, to organize the boxes of clippings from the championship season, and to recycle half of the basement! It is a time to nurture friendships, read books, and to learn to play my old piano. It is a time to love and be loved.

It is also a time to recognize that the innocence of my childhood must not be confused with the innocence of time and place. Growing up in Medfield during the fifties and sixties, I was protected from much that is ugly in the world. Masked by the sameness of its population, biases and prejudices lay dormant but not forgotten. Sexism wasn't challenged, it was a way of life; girls wore ruffles and boys played ball. Religious intolerance was hidden as we worshipped behind closed doors on Sunday; there was never a joining together in communal prayer. There was no synagogue or mosque. Racial tension is not a problem when a town remains lily white. As my experience in life broadened, I became more aware of the stereotypes that had been quietly engraved on my subconscious.

This struck me, when, after years of vacationing on Cape Cod, we decided to watch the annual Gay Parade in Provincetown, a yearly event sponsored by the large gay community there. It was intended to be a festive affair, but I viewed it with many mixed emotions. As costumed gays, lesbians, and transvestites made their way along the narrow streets of Provincetown, I suddenly spotted among them a young man from Southwick. At once, I was overcome by a kind of unsettled sadness. Why do our young people, homosexual or not, rebel more than they really want to in their search for acceptance. Are they expressing something real within themselves, or is it their way of holding up a mirror to the fears, intolerance, and ignorance they see in society at large. Perhaps I am my brother's keeper.

Writing this book has given me time for personal reflection that everyday life rarely affords. I see more clearly now which of the values and convictions I was raised with are indispensable and which are not. "Family values" can't be carved in stone. They are more like the pliable threads upon which a tapestry is woven; they support the changing colors and patterns of our lives. The lives of my children, their problems and triumphs, conspire to keep me focused on the present and distract me from trying to find hard and fast rules for my life or anyone else's. Armed with the past, renewed in the moment, and challenged by the future, I am proud of the lives my children are making for themselves. As I reflect on how these new patterns will be woven into our family story, I am confident that the loom on which Den's and my labor is crafted will be strong enough to support the life fabric of our children.

Afterwords

★ *RACHEL*

Rebecca is never one to brag or put herself first. However, I do remember one occasion when my sister actually exhibited her knowledge of her own "greatness."

We were sitting around in our bedroom, which we shared only because it was the biggest room in the house, and my mother wouldn't let me have it otherwise. Anyway, while discussing boys and clothes, the topic of conversation drifted toward basketball. At the time I was a sophomore in high school playing junior varsity basketball, and she was an eighth grader. I told her that she was going to have to work really hard to make varsity as a freshman. She told me, "Yeah, I know. But I'm gonna make varsity anyway. Who else do they have to play center?"

I was surprised because that's not something that Rebecca would ordinarily say. I told her there were several candidates for the position, and we really didn't need her that much. She responded, "Rach, I'm gonna make varsity and I'm going to play a lot." Deep down inside, I knew that she was right, but I felt I had to make her doubt herself somehow. A year later I was congratulating her for setting a school record for the most points in a game scored by a freshman.

I can recall going shopping for school clothes and every time I picked out something to wear, Rebecca picked out the same thing. As a young girl, trying to establish my own identity, I used to get very frustrated and angry when Rebecca did this. On a few occasions, I purposely picked out ugly outfits just so my mom would buy them for her. Then, of course, I picked something else and had Mom buy that for me. I didn't realize or appreciate then what it meant to be an older sister. It was something I just always took for granted. I don't anymore.

If I could have one wish, it would be that on my wedding day, I would look at my fiancé and myself in the mirror and the reflection there would be of the love that I have seen between my parents. Whether it is seeing them hug and kiss in the kitchen, or snoring out of sync together on the couch, they are the vision I carry with me as I start a life of my own.

When asked if I am a "Lobo, too," I simply smile and say "Yes."

Everything else just takes care of itself.

★ *JASON*

"So, how does it feel to be Rebecca Lobo's brother?"

"Can she beat you at one-on-one?"

"How tall is she in comparison to you?"

"What is she doing now?"

"How is your mom doing? She's in our prayers."

"You must hear these questions all the time."

A day does not seem complete without one of these questions or comments. Although the inquiries are usually the same, I never tire of them. It's easy talking about those you love. Plus, you meet so many interesting people.

The summer after my mother's bout with cancer provided a chance for Rachel, Rebecca, and me to get together with a number of my friends at The Cellar in Hartford. Rebecca asked me to get her a Coca-Cola, soda glass, and straw to expertly disguise what she was really drinking, while Rachel was content to share pitchers of beer with my friends. She's a clever one, that Rebecca. (By the way, Mom, I actually had more than one beer at the high school party you mentioned. But I still learned my lesson.) The drive home also provided us our first opportunity to talk about what our mother had been through. I had seen its effect on my father and mother, but was unaware of the depth it touched both sisters. I had never connected my mother's illness with my own health. For good reason, my sisters had.

We talked then about the importance of our parents in our lives and our fear of losing them. We compared our self-images and feelings toward each other. Perhaps for the first time I realized that my "baby" sisters had grown into complex and wondrous women. The beer also helped Rachel demonstrate her love to my parents by waking them and sobbing her expressions of affection to them in their room. Rebecca and I were unable to appreciate her full litany as we were clutching each other in the hall, doubled over with suppressed laughter and giggles. "Do you think they know she's been drinking?"

My sisters are now two of my closest friends. As Rachel lives two-and-a-half-hours away and Rebecca is everywhere else, they are the two friends I probably see the least. Yet when we are together, a closeness exists at an elemental level that I am unable to describe.

So, how does it feel to be Rebecca Lobo's big brother? The same as it feels to be Rachel Lobo's brother and Dennis and RuthAnn Lobo's son. Constantly teased and absolutely wonderful. Can she beat me at one-on-one? No, but now I announce to the neighborhood if I beat her at Horse. How tall is she in comparison to me? She is approximately seven inches shorter, hence the one-on-one superiority. (Right, Becca?) What is she doing now? Enjoying her life to the fullest and caring for those around her. How is my Mom? If this Afterword doesn't end up on the editing room floor and you are actually reading this sentence, I assume you've read the book first. I hope you've ascertained that Mom is doing great and is almost as busy as Rebecca. Never underestimate the power of prayer.

And though I do hear these questions all the time, I hope people never stop asking them.